NIPS & TUCKS

Everything You Must Know

Before Having

Cosmetic Surgery

• • •

BY DIANA BARRY

Publisher: W. Quay Hays
Editor: Peter Hoffman
Art Director: Susan Anson
Projects Manager: Trudihope Schlomowitz
Production Director: Nadeen Torio
Color and Pre-press Manager: Bill Castillo
Color and Pre-press Director: Gaston Moraga
Production Artist: Phillis Stacy
Production Assistants: Tom Archibeque, Alan Peak
Copy Editors: Lynette Padwa, George Garrigues

Cover photo: © Mark Davison/Tony Stone Images
Illustrations: Shirley H. Coleman

For information:
General Publishing Group, Inc.
2701 Ocean Park Boulevard
Santa Monica, CA 90405

Library of Congress Cataloging-in-Publication Data

Barry, Diana
       Nips & tucks : everything you must know before having cosmetic
surgery / by Diana Barry.
              p.   cm.
       Includes index.
       ISBN 1-881649-93-8
       1. Surgery, Plastic—Popular works. 2. Surgery, Plastic—
Psychological aspects.   I. Title.
       RD119.B32 1996
       617.9'5—dc20   96-2521
                                                                           CIP

Printed in the USA by RR Donnelley & Sons Company
10 9 8 7 6 5 4 3 2 1

GENERAL PUBLISHING GROUP
Los Angeles

Table of Contents

...

Acknowledgments

• • •

With deepest appreciation:

Dr. Anthony Sokol

Dr. Gary Lask

Dr. Robert Kotler

Dr. Ronald Moy

Dr. David Hopp

Dr. Athleo Cambre

Dr. Stephen Bosniak

Dr. Miriam Zilkha

Dr. Randolph Sherman

Dr. Sidney Sonenblum

Dr. Barbara Biggs

Pauline Sugine

Maria Teresa Boni

Chris Price

Quay Hays

Sharon Hays

Susan Anson

Peter Hoffman

Lori Rick

Shirley Coleman

Foreword

• • •

I have had the pleasure of reviewing this book on cosmetic surgery by Diana Barry. This is one of the finest books written for prospective patients on this subject.

Ms. Barry is well qualified to write this text. Although trained as a make-up artist, she learned early on that a successful recovery from plastic surgery consists of many other areas of support besides make-up, including counseling, information and reassurance. She has provided a text of immense importance, which serves to inform the prospective patient about the journey through cosmetic surgery. The book also describes a method to enable the patient to best prepare him or herself for the procedure, both mentally and physically. This will make the operation safer and improve the patient's response.

The operative and postoperative courses of the various cosmetic procedures are beautifully described. This will help reduce any fear and anxiety that may occur during the period preceding surgery, as well as the stress which can occur during the postoperative period, when the patient may encounter swelling, discomfort, discoloration and dissatisfaction, addressing the issues in clear, understandable language that is both reassuring and informative. Ms. Barry's text allows her to personally hold each and every reader's hand through the entire procedure of cosmetic surgery.

As a surgeon, I realize it is sometimes difficult to know how much information to impart to a patient in order to assist him or her with a decision to undergo cosmetic surgery. Some patients will require only the basic facts of the procedure, its risks, goals and complications. Others may need a much more detailed description. This book will assist both the patient and the cosmetic surgeon by providing additional sources of information. I recommend it to each person contemplating plastic surgery as well as every cosmetic surgeon. As a doctor who specializes in cosmetic surgery, I have found the book provided a new and different perspective that will benefit my practice.

—*Anthony B. Sokol, M.D., F.A.C.S.*
Diplomate, American Board of Plastic Surgery
Chief, Division of Plastic Surgery,
Cedars-Sinai Medical Center

Preface

. . .

My involvement with plastic surgery began because of a tragedy. My father was one of the first people shot in the 1965 Watts riots. A double-barreled shotgun was placed against the driver's window of his car and fired directly at his head, blowing close to half his face away.

I remember seeing him lying in the hospital, unrecognizable and near death, while doctors and plastic surgeons demanded to see any and every rendering that existed of my dad…photographs, portraits, home movies. The walls of the operating room were covered with his photos, as skilled plastic and reconstructive surgeons began their magic. First, synthetic bone structure to duplicate his facial shape. Dental reconstruction. Endless reconstructive procedures. And amazingly enough, in lieu of skin grafts his double chin was lifted up and secured to the areas that had been blown away.

After a long and traumatic recovery my father miraculously looked like his old self. With the exception of some minor scarring that eventually nearly disappeared, he was very definitely wearing his own face. So here I am, a passionate witness to the wonders of plastic surgery.

I am not a doctor. I don't pretend to be a medical authority in any form. My work has been in the worlds of fashion, beauty and the theatre. I was a successful photo-model for several years, with many magazine covers to my credit—including *Vogue* and *Harper's Bazaar*—and later was a fashion director of Neiman Marcus, Beverly Hills. I've acted in film, TV, commercials and on the stage throughout my lifetime. I realized I could help post-surgical patients by teaching them all of the photographic and theatrical makeup tricks I had learned along the way. These were women who had had elective surgeries (primarily face-lifts), as well as women who had undergone reconstructive surgeries following strokes and traumatic accidents.

I have worked for some of the best plastic surgeons in Beverly Hills and Los Angeles for years, and this book is a collective account of what I have observed to be predictable and normal reactions that most women will experience, particularly during their first six to eight weeks of recovery from surgery.

Obviously, experiencing an elective face-lift doesn't remotely resemble the trauma of recovering from accidents or medical reconstructive surgeries. However, I have learned that the most difficult part of having a face-lift is the three weeks after the surgery, mainly because most plastic surgeons and their office staff play down the postsurgical symptoms of recovery.

Who knows why? Perhaps it's because they realize that the distortion, memory loss, depression, lack of energy and so forth that many patients experience will usually pass within several weeks. Perhaps they don't discuss this recovery period in any depth because they fear it would frighten the patient away from the surgery. Most offices provide printed material that mentions—superficially—the possibility of two or three days of depression, some swelling and a little fatigue.

Well, I don't know about you, but my attitude is: Let me know *precisely* what to expect. If it doesn't happen, wonderful! If it does happen, I won't feel like the unfortunate exception, frightened and unnecessarily anxious.

This book will help you understand what you can expect during your recovery period. Not everyone will experience these reactions. Occasionally, someone sails through the entire experience effortlessly and beautifully. Most people, however, have some temporary complaints, and my hope is that this book will prevent you from feeling victimized by a lack of knowledge on the subject.

—Diana Barry

With love

to the memories of my father, Sam Newman,

and Dr. Giovanni Boni

Part One:
The Face-Lift

CHAPTER ONE

Why a Face-Lift?

• • •

The bottom line is: *do this surgery for yourself...only for yourself.* Your face-lift will not change your life, solve your problems, fix your failing marriage or make you feel 25 again. Most plastic surgeons explain that a successful face-lift will make you look beautifully "rested and refreshed." That's quite true; it more or less cleans up the haggard look that comes with having survived real life for X amount of years. A face-lift will also eliminate loose skin around the neck, jowls and upper and lower eye areas.

Do yourself a favor and don't go to see your doctor with an attitude of talking him into giving you an overkill face-lift, one that's pulled so taut that no character is left in the face. You don't want to look like some bizarre doll. You just want to look like the most beautiful natural version of yourself. This means you must insist that several soft, natural expression lines remain on your finished face. You don't want people looking at you and saying, "What a beautiful face-job"; you want them to say, "You look beautiful." So, believe me, get that image of a fantasy-face without a single line on it out of your mind right now. It's a dead giveaway of a face-job, and who needs that?

Another thing you must realize up front is that almost no one is born with absolutely symmetrical features. You should not expect to emerge from your face-lift with a "perfect face." In my opinion, a face-lift is like everything else in life: It's a trade-off. You will most certainly look remarkably better after surgery, but you will never look perfect.

It's not that your surgeon won't try everything within his technical and artistic abilities to achieve perfection. But no matter how brilliant your doctor is, the fact remains that an enormous amount of your finished face-lift is determined by your own body, skin type, skin damage and individual systemic behavior.

Additionally, some people heal much faster than others and experience less discomfort and fewer problems. It's systemic and unpredictable. So don't decide that just because your girlfriend looked and felt fabulous three weeks after her surgery, you will too. The reality is that you may love your face two-and-a-half weeks after surgery, or it may take you four or six or eight weeks to really feel happy with what you see and begin to have a normal energy level again. The body will move at its own pace. It will heal itself as evenly and as well as it's capable.

Of course, there always exists the possibility that your doctor actually will not remove enough skin to satisfy you, or that you'll be unhappy with the "surgical look" of something. This is a completely separate issue from your own skin characteristics and systemic makeup, and you'll need to discuss it very openly with your doctor. In all fairness, you will not be able to accurately judge a problem in need of correction until at least the eighth or ninth week after surgery, because the normal swelling, shifting, thickening and pulling of areas will not settle down until then. You may believe you have a problem when in reality it's just the normal healing process that will correct itself with time. However, speak to your doctor as soon as you see anything that bothers you. It's part of his job to provide you with that peace of mind.

If there is indeed a surgical problem you are unhappy about, you must plainly voice your dissatisfaction to your doctor and demand a surgical correction if it's possible. Your surgeon may explain to you, for example, "If I pulled this area tighter, it would have created unattractive lines in the adjoining area." You don't know why he made the choices he did until you give him the opportunity to explain his judgment. Often the doctor is right. Sometimes, however, he just didn't remove enough skin, or something is disturbingly uneven. If it is at all possible, a credible plastic surgeon will not hesitate to correct these problems for you at his own expense.

A postsurgical recovery period of at least three months is usually required for most touch-ups or corrections. Some procedures require even longer periods between surgeries; your doctor will advise you on scheduling. Listen to him! It's unsafe to reoperate too soon on an area, and you'll only run into more problems if you proceed before the appropriate time. It's better to be a little patient and end up with a face you love.

So, to repeat, expect the Desired Trade-Off: You *will* look remarkably better.

Don't go looking for every detail to be perfect. The body doesn't usually work that way. It's unrealistic and you'll only end up driving your doctor and, more important, yourself nuts!

CHAPTER TWO

Choosing Your Doctor

• • •

When choosing a plastic surgeon, there is one cardinal rule: Shop around. Take consultations with at least three doctors. Consultations usually run around $150 and up, and are often credited toward the total fees of the office you finally choose. Spend the extra money auditioning these doctors. Your surgery is a large financial investment and, more important, you'll have to live with your new face for a very long time. It's absolutely essential that you feel secure, confident and personally comfortable with the doctor you choose. The actual cost of a full face-lift without any additional procedures usually runs from $5,000 to $15,000. Fees for lab tests and anesthesiology costs will be separate. *Never* choose a plastic surgeon simply because his fee is lower. A discount fee may very well leave you with a bargain-basement face.

Most women go to doctors who have worked on their friends, which is actually a rather intelligent approach. At least you're able to see for yourself if your friend's face-lift seems natural and artistically appealing. She'll also be able to tell you how available the doctor was throughout the event, and to rate the overall tone and cooperation of the office staff. Word-of-mouth recommendations are extremely useful, especially if they are rave reviews. They should be included on your list to research and interview.

I would never choose a plastic surgeon who is big on media advertising. The very best doctors are so busy with their word-of-mouth success that they don't need to place ads in magazines, etc. (This is not to be confused with an actual article a publication may choose to run about an outstanding doctor.) Many women will select a doctor they've seen interviewed on a television show. This can be tricky, because many of these doctors hire public-relations firms to create high profiles, and they are not necessarily your safest choice. Of course, some of the very best surgeons have been on the air as well. The only way you can determine the right surgeon is to do your homework.

Contact the American Board of Plastic and Reconstructive Surgeons, the American Academy of Facial Plastic Surgery, the American Academy of Cosmetic Surgery or the American Society for Dermatologic Surgery. Ask them for a list of doctors in the city where you want to have your surgery. Request the surgeons' resume from their individual offices. Research your doctor; the more you know about his credentials, the safer you'll feel. Your choice of doctor needs to be a result of intelligent and thorough research on your part. When you consider a face-lift, the physician's credentials are your primary focus. Obviously, a Board Certified Plastic Surgeon is always a safe choice. *You must be absolutely certain that if your doctor isn't a Board Certified Plastic Surgeon, he is a current member of the American Academy of Facial Plastic Surgery.*

Other specialists should be considered for specific procedures that are not face-lifts. Many excellent ear, nose and throat surgeons may also be some of your best possible choices. A top ophthalmic surgeon could be a good choice for eyelid surgery. Certainly the best dermatologists are a smart option for liposuction and line-filler procedures, such as collagen and fat transplants. I would choose a top dermatologist to perform any type of chemical peel, dermabrasion or laser surgery.

Your choice of doctor ultimately will be based on two factors: experience and specialized skills, and your personal rapport with him.

The most important factor you must establish with your doctor is open, comfortable and clear communication. One of the worst mistakes anyone can make is simply to say to a plastic surgeon, "You have carte blanche, just make me beautiful." You must have a reasonably clear idea of how you want to look, and you must express this during your consultation. The doctor may also have some suggestions you'll want to consider, but don't walk in vague and vulnerable. Too many bad surprises can occur when you hand a doctor total artistic freedom.

This type of disaster nearly happened to a close friend of mine, a very beautiful former cover girl who, when she was in her middle 50s, took consultations with several Beverly Hills surgeons. She very succinctly explained to them that she wanted to end up "looking like myself, with no great alterations to my features, but hopefully eight to ten years younger." A very reasonable remark. One doctor quipped back, "Look at it this way: When you're asleep and under my knife, I'll do what I consider will look good, and that's what you'll wake up with."

Wrong! Wrong! Wrong!

Forget this doctor! Of course, any doctor will do what he considers medically and artistically correct. But it's *your face*. You, not the doctor, will have to live in it and with it. It's part of his job to work *with you* to create a final result that you both agree can be achieved. Be very sure that the doctor you are interviewing is 100 percent willing to answer all your technical and artistic questions to a degree that will satisfy you. If the doctor is not willing to communicate with you on this level, you have the wrong doctor. Keep looking.

Granted, you are not taking a consultation about surgery relating to a terminal illness. You are discussing a face-lift. But make no mistake, elective cosmetic surgery is not a minor procedure. The amount of anesthesia that you will be given (usually three to five hours for a face-lift with no additional procedures) indicates that this is a serious, although not particularly dangerous, surgery. The trauma of having your face cut into, muscles sutured, proportions resculptured, possible implants, bone work, repositioning of skin and so forth is far from minor. None of it feels hideous, so don't get scared! But don't ever trust a doctor who declares, "Oh, it's nothing, believe me." A face-lift is real surgery. It's not a nip and a tuck and then you can go tap dancing.

Don't completely count on a doctor's statement that you can be back at work or your everyday life looking and feeling absolutely normal in two weeks. This seems to happen to only about 50 percent of face-lift patients. The other 50 percent take a bit longer to normalize. You may be able to get back to work in two weeks, but more likely you'll experience some serious fatigue each afternoon and evening until the end of the third or fourth week. It usually takes eight full weeks to completely regain your normal energy level, just as it does after most surgeries. Many women, however, begin to feel a decent, sustained energy level and to love the way they look between the third and fourth week after surgery. Frankly, you're usually too swollen and distorted to like the way you look until the end of the third postsurgical week, but I'll get into that subject in Chapter 5.

I recently received a telephone call from a well-known soap opera actress who was in tears because her doctor assured her that she would be able to go in front of the camera two weeks after her face-lift. Well, two weeks had arrived, and her incision lines were still raised and thick and red around her eyes—a typical situation. I get crazed with doctors who tell women they'll be gorgeous and active in two weeks. A charming bedside manner is always nice, but find a doctor who will level with you. No one can precisely second-guess your body's individual pace of recovery. And a word to actors planning a face-lift: Don't expect to be "camera-ready" for close-ups until the end of the third or fourth week after surgery, and that's cutting it short.

As with all relationships, communication with your doctor is a two-way street. Doctors are human; they have their good days and bad days. Approach them as people. I will never understand patients who are afraid to openly express themselves to their doctors. Help them all you can by answering every question honestly, and supply them with any additional information you consider medically or personally pertinent, such as any real fears regarding your surgery, severe emotional traumas you are going through and so on.

Also, make sure they know that you expect them to be there for you before surgery, during surgery and after surgery at your check-ups. Some doctors disappear after the actual surgery is completed and the check is cashed. They will occasionally pop in for a two-minute postsurgical look-see, then leave you to deal with nurses and office staff, all of whom might be thoroughly competent. That's not good enough. Insist on knowing that the surgeon you choose will be available for a reasonable (not insane) number of postsurgical questions. To save everyone's time, have a written list of specific questions with you.

You've paid a lot of money for this face-lift. That entitles you to presurgical, surgical and postsurgical care by the doctor. There's a difference between being a reasonably demanding patient and being needy and neurotic. You're *allowed* to be reasonably demanding, which means if you have valid questions, get them answered.

CHAPTER THREE

Before Your Surgery

• • •

When I go in for any form of elective medical procedure, I become as disciplined as a professional athlete. I want to give myself every possible advantage to heal quickly and beautifully.

About two weeks before surgery I begin taking a homeopathic remedy called Arnica Montana 200X once a day. Homeopathic remedies are natural and contain absolutely no drugs, and Arnica can be safely taken by anyone. This particular remedy is a big favorite among professional athletes because it reduces bruising in the most remarkable way. If you take Arnica before your surgery, and continue it once a day for two weeks afterward, you'll still have some bruising, but it will be much less than normal for your system, and it will disappear more quickly.

There's a technique to taking homeopathic remedies that must be rigidly followed. You must not eat, drink or smoke anything 20 minutes before or after taking the remedy. If you do, the remedy will not work. The best solution is to take the Arnica upon rising each morning, and then just wait the full 20 minutes before coffee and breakfast. Arnica costs less than $10 for a one-ounce bottle, which is all you'll need. It comes in the form of small, sweet, white pellets that you place under the tongue and let dissolve. You must never touch the pellets with your hands; they will neutralize and not work properly. Instead, roll six pellets directly into the bottle cap and throw them under your tongue from the cap. Never take Arnica in a strength other than 200X or 5c for cosmetic surgery. If you are taking a 5c strength, you will take 3 pellets instead of 6 pellets.

Many cities have homeopathic pharmacies. If you can't find one, you can always have the remedies shipped to you.[1]

A good two weeks before surgery I also take at least 200 mg of vitamin C (you may need to reduce the amount if it upsets your stomach), bio-flavonoids and Rutin to combat bruising, vitamin K to help control blood clotting and a really good multivitamin that includes minerals such as B-complex, zinc and vitamin E. My presurgery training regimen also includes the elimination of all rich foods and alcohol, and I flush my system out with considerably more water than I normally drink. None of these suggestions is mandatory. But my attitude is, why not go in for your surgery in the strongest and cleanest shape possible?

At some point before surgery it is essential that you stop drinking alcohol and smoking. Your doctor and the anesthesiologist will give you this information. If taken 8 to 10 hours before surgery, alcohol makes anesthesia dangerous. Smoking significantly retards the healing process in the face. Never trust a doctor who tells you that it is okay to smoke up until your surgery date and immediately afterward. I've seen some horrendous permanent results on the faces of women who refused to quit smoking before their surgery. Most offices will suggest quitting smoking a minimum of a week to 10 days before surgery. If it were me, I'd quit a minimum of three weeks prior to surgery and not smoke again until at least three weeks afterward. I know how incredibly hard this is for longtime smokers, but why risk the possibility of permanent problems? Discuss with your doctor precisely when he feels it's necessary for you to quit smoking and—please—do yourself an enormous favor and listen to him.

About two weeks before surgery your doctor will require you to have blood tests and lab work done. Don't be surprised if an AIDS test is included in the workup; many doctors are insisting on it now.

Your doctor may also suggest presurgical supplements such as vitamin K. You must stop all aspirin-containing products at this time. Aspirin will cause more bruising and perhaps even bleeding, and it will delay your recovery. The chart on page 25 lists aspirin-containing products that you must avoid.

[1]The Santa Monica Drug Company, 629 Broadway, Santa Monica, CA 90401 (310-395-1131). Drug Stop 22, 8021 Melrose Avenue, Los Angeles, CA 90046 (1-800-248-9030). Capitol Drugs, 8578 Santa Monica Blvd., West Hollywood, California 90069 (1-800-858-8833). All of the above stores will ship your orders to you via U.P.S.

One of your most crucial sessions will be with the anesthesiologist. He will ask you very specific questions about your medical history and about your allergies and reactions to certain drugs. Be absolutely precise about every single answer and piece of information you give the anesthesiologist. If you're not sure of an answer, research it and advise him of the correct information. It's imperative that you are never vague with the anesthesiologist.

There are some remarkable new drugs available that leave you much less groggy after surgery than used to be the case. Ask your anesthesiologist exactly what you should expect in this regard. Also, if you have any urinary retention problems, you'll need to discuss the choice of antinausea medication because such medication has occasionally been known to slow the urinary functions. The anesthesiologist will give you itemized medications, with instructions, to be taken the night before and sometimes even the morning of surgery, with one tiny swallow of water. *Otherwise, absolutely no food or water is allowed after midnight the night before or the morning of surgery.*

I urge you to openly discuss fears you may have about anesthesia with the anesthesiologist. It's part of his job to deal with it and provide you with medical reassurance.

The office will supply you with detailed instructions about hair washing, presurgical food and liquid intake restrictions, the type of clothing you should arrive in and medication you will be taking. Also included will be a list of medications you absolutely must not take before surgery, such as aspirin.

During this period you should arrange for an aftercare facility. It's a terrible idea to even think of going home after a face-lift. You need to be monitored professionally for the first night following your surgery at the very least. Aftercare facilities range from simple and clean to chic and extravagant. The price is usually $350 to $500 a night plus supply costs. Most women stay one to three nights, and some stay up to two weeks or longer, until their "distorted period" has subsided, although this is not medically necessary. The aftercare people will pick you up after surgery, drive you to the facility (don't expect to be too awake or peppy for this particular ride), settle you into your bed and begin your care.

A good aftercare facility will monitor you at least once each hour, perhaps more, depending on your age and general state of health. The staff will medicate you according to your doctor's instructions, feed you the appropriate soft foods and liquids and make certain that you're as comfortable as possible. If a nurse is not in to see you at least once every hour, raise holy hell! Demand the attention. Insist they call your doctor for you, if it comes to that.

The first afternoon and evening following surgery you can feel rather rocky and groggy. Some women experience nausea, but it's usually gone by evening if not before. The nurses will help you through any problems.

You'll have a helmet dressing covering the entire top and back of your head, with extended bandages down over the ears and secured under your chin to hold everything nicely in place. Some women feel slightly claustrophobic in this high-pressure helmet dressing. Don't panic! Try to readjust your thinking and know that it is necessary and may be replaced with a lightweight dressing when you see your doctor for your first postoperative checkup the day after surgery. The lighter bandages will stay on for another two days. Some doctors may place one drain on either side of the neck to avoid the possibility of bleeding problems. The drains can be rather uncomfortable, but they too are slipped out the day following surgery.

The good news is that you are not in pain. The interesting thing about face-lifts, eye-jobs and forehead-lifts is that although you experience some odd and uncomfortable temporary sensations, such as numbness and swelling, there's never any remarkable pain. Your doctor will prescribe medication to take the edge off the discomfort. Some women don't even need to use it. If you want a painkiller, take it; it will help you ignore the momentary annoyance. If you are feeling a definite and obvious pain anywhere under your dressings, call the nurse immediately and have her contact your doctor at once. It could be an indication of blood clots that would require instant medical attention.

The aftercare staff will drive you to and from your doctor's office for as many postsurgical checkups as you require during your aftercare stay.

Family and friends are usually allowed to visit you at the aftercare facility, following your completed arrival and medical monitoring. Some aftercare houses will even provide meals and sleeping accommodations for friends and relatives.

Believe me, they're the place to be following your surgery. If you don't want to go to an aftercare facility, hire a private nurse to stay with you at home for one to three nights. You'll be thankful for the necessary and professional assistance!

AN ASPIRIN DIRECTORY

These common, brand-name prescription and over-the-counter drugs contain aspirin. It's necessary to stop using them at least two weeks prior to surgery and for one week after. They can cause bleeding and bruising. This list does not include any generic preparations sold under store brands or other names.

Alka-Seltzer tablets
Alka-Seltzer Plus cold medicine
Anacin capsules and tablets
APC tablets
APC with Butalbital tablets
APC with Codeine Tabloid brand
Anacin Maximum Strength
Arthritis Pain Formula (Anacin)
Arthritis Strength Bufferin
Ascriptin
Aspergum
Aspirin suppositories
Bayer Aspirin
Bayer Children's Chewable Aspirin
Bayer Children's Cold Tablets
Bayer Timed-Released Aspirin
Buff-A Comp tablets
Bufferin
Cama Inlay-Tabs
Cetased, Improved
Congespirin
Coricidin D decongestant tablets
Coricidin for children
Coricidin Medilets tablets
    for children
Coricidin tablets
Darvon with A.S.A.
Darvon-N with A.S.A.
Dristan decongestant
Ecotrin tablets
Empirin
Empirin with Codeine
Emprazil tablets

Emprazil-C tablets En Tab
Excedrin
Extra-Strength Bufferin
Fiorinal
Fiorinal with Codeine
4-Way Cold Tablets
Gemnisyn
Goody's Headache Powders
Midol
Momentum Muscular
    Backache Formula
Norgesic
Norgesic Forte
Norwich Aspirin
Pabirin buffered tablets
Panalgesic
Percodan and Percodan-
    Demi tablets
Quiet World Analgesic /
    Sleeping Aid
Robaxisal tablets
SK-65 Compound
St. Joseph Aspirin for Children
Sine-Off Sinus Medicine
Supac
Synalgos capsules
Synalgos-DC capsule
Triaminicin tablets
Vanquish
Verin
Viro-Med tablets
Zorprin

Source: *Physicians' Desk Reference and Physicians' Desk Reference for Non-prescription Drugs.*

CHAPTER FOUR

The Lower Face-Lift

• • •

APPROXIMATE COST: $4,400–$7,000

There may be additional charges for surgical facilities and anesthesia. Be sure to request this information.

THE SURGERY

The surgery takes approximately three hours. There are normally four people in the operating room with you: the surgeon, the anesthesiologist and two surgical nurses.

Anesthesia is most commonly administered intravenously. A local anesthetic is used simultaneously to numb the operative area. This is called intravenous sedation or local standby anesthesia. An anesthesiologist or nurse anesthetist is utilized to assure that the patient is comfortable and that the procedure is carried out safely. Some plastic surgeons prefer general anesthesia to I.V. sedation. They feel that it gives them better control and that the patient will have a more speedy recovery. Although the procedure is controversial, the patient may actually receive less medication this way.

Your doctor will decide which type of anesthesia is best for you. The anesthetic drugs that are used today wear off very quickly, which is a definite advantage. Medication is used with both types of anesthetic to minimize postoperative nausea and coughing that would cause discomfort and lead to bleeding.

The neck is infiltrated with Xylocaine and Epinephrine. Throughout the procedure the Xylocaine and Epinephrine are used even if the patient is asleep, as these drugs cause the blood vessels and tissues to constrict, thus reducing bleeding that would interfere with the surgeon's ability to judge the anatomy and surgical decisions he'll be making.

The procedure is basically composed of three steps:

1. The removal of fat beneath the jaw.

2. The tightening of tissues deep to the skin.

3. The removal of excess skin with closure.

An incision line is made behind the chin pad (three to four millimeters long) and a small hose is inserted for liposuction in the neck. Special attention is given to the fat pads at the jowl line. If the patient has cords in the front of the neck, the cords are sutured together to give a smooth contour to the neck. If this is necessary, the incision is extended to 1-1/2 millimeters.

Incisions are made in the ear area, preferably just under the sideburn so the sideburn will cover the scar. An incision is then made inside the ear, around the earlobe, up behind the ear to the center muscle, and then diagonally back into the scalp behind the ear. A word to male patients: The scalp incision often looks cleaner when it's run just along the bottom hairline, rather than diagonally into the hair. This is not a good idea for women, as it would show when you wore your hair up.

A dissection is then made just beneath the skin and skin fat, to the fold between the lip and the cheek, and to the mid-line of the neck. Great care is taken by the surgeon to avoid any damage to nerves that supply sensation to the ear and to muscles that provide animation to the face. Although these areas can be injured, a careful surgeon usually avoids any damage.

Following this dissection the skin is raised and the flat sheet of muscle that encompasses either side of the neck (the platysmal muscle) is elevated from the underlying tissue. The platysmal muscle, also known as the SMAS, is actually a muscle system running from just under your ear, down over the jaw, down the side of the neck to the top of the breastbone. This thin superficial muscle system is pulled backward in order to provide a deep support to the tissue of the face, particularly around the jaw, and then sutured to the tissue just under the skin behind the ear. The fat overlying that area is removed to give a sleek, clean look. Six to eight sutures are placed down either side of the neck to secure the SMAS back in that area.

A considerable amount of time is then given to coagulate all of the blood vessels. Any bleeding in the face can result in later problems, and every effort is sought to control this.

The extra skin is carefully trimmed so it won't cause any wrinkles or pulling. The sutures that are used for most of the pulling are behind the ear. The cheek skin is also pulled and secured to the ear. Stitching is done with care in order to minimize scarring.

Drains may be placed in the neck in order to siphon off any oozing that may occur in the first 24 hours. The drains are removed the following day.

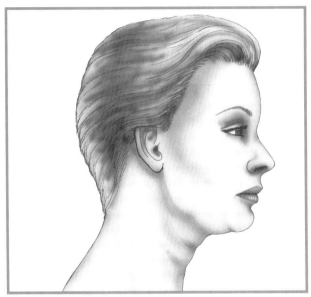

Prior to surgery, drooping muscles around the mouth, sagging jowls and a neck with loose skin are all prominently visible.

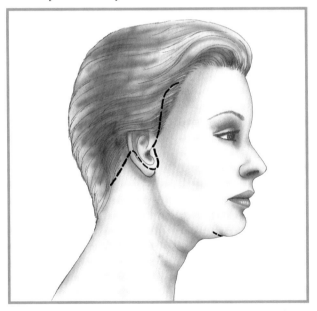

An incision is made behind the chin pad for liposuction. Incisions are hidden within or just under the sideburn, inside the ear, around the earlobe, up behind the ear to the center muscle and diagonally into the scalp behind the ear.

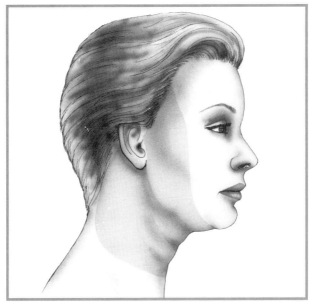

The shaded area shows where the skin will be dissected and raised to allow for tightening of the SMAS.

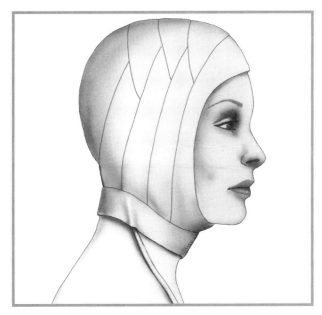

The head is bandaged following surgery. Drains may be placed on either side of the neck to drain blood.

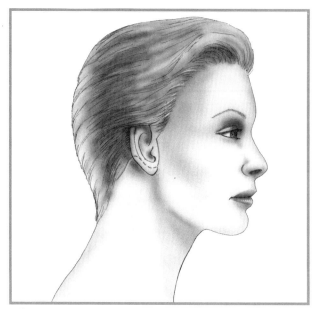

The postoperative face and neck is remarkably firm and sleek.

CHAPTER FIVE

What to Expect When You Come Home

• • •

You're finally home. Basically, you look like a Pillsbury doughboy who's been in an auto wreck. Between bouts of crying, shock, depression and exhaustion, you're staring at this unrecognizable face, trying to comprehend why you did this to yourself.

Do not panic! It's only a temporary state—it will all go away! And you will actually start to fall in love with the way you look by two or three weeks post-surgery.

I believe that the greatest oversight by most plastic surgeons is their failure to furnish the patient with a detailed explanation of symptoms they should expect to experience during the normal healing process. Too many doctor's offices assume an attitude of, "You're just more sensitive than most people," or, "Well, gee, it must be you—most people aren't upset or concerned," or, "You're just overreacting. Get a grip on yourself."

I don't know why these particular offices choose to deal with the postoperative period this way, but I consider it a monumental disservice to the patient. It's entirely possible that occasionally a person will be more sensitive than others. It's also possible that some of you luckier people will only experience very mild versions of the healing process. But the majority of you can expect the following normal symptoms during your first few weeks of recovery.

The first two to three weeks after surgery are commonly referred to as the "Distorted Period"…and when you're in it, you'll know why. You will probably be given steroids for swelling, but some swelling is still very likely. The surprising thing about the swelling that follows facial surgery is that it never looks symmetrical. One cheek can look much larger than the other. One eye can seem totally different in shape than the other. Many women are frightened that their doctor "didn't make them even." *Relax!* In 99 percent of the cases, your surgeon made you as even as possible. What you're looking at now is the postsurgical swelling, which distorts everything. And don't be the least bit surprised if the swelling shifts all over your face the first two to three weeks, because it most likely will.

In some areas, such as under the chin, the swelling will usually seem puffy and rock solid. Again, don't assume the surgeon didn't lift that area to your satisfaction. It will all soften up and then tighten up to where you hoped it would be. Also, unattractive ridges or tucks may appear on areas of your cheeks or around the mouth. It's just swelling that will disappear and smooth out over the next few weeks. Not everyone develops these uneven areas, but if you do, just know that it's temporary and will all flatten out in a little while.

Sometimes the swelling is so hard in spots that the doctor will send you for a few ultrasound treatments. This is extremely useful in breaking up stubborn swelling, and the patient experiences relief very quickly.

The glossy, masklike appearance that's obvious and temporary after a face-lift is also due to swelling. By the fourth week most women adore their faces because the distorted period has passed, but there remains just enough swelling to plump out all the natural lines. Enjoy this stage while you can because as the swelling continues to disappear your natural lines will softly begin to return. Be thankful that they do. You don't want to be stuck with that masklike face for the next several years. We've all seen women who have been surgically pulled too tight, and it's a horror show. Interestingly enough, the majority of those women have insisted their surgeon do this to them. *Huge mistake—don't you make it!*

Although you will probably begin to love your face by the third or fourth week post-op, there is no way you can begin to judge your final results until the end of the eighth week. By then the obvious swelling has disappeared, although the healing process will continue internally for several more months.

Most bruising goes through a predictable pattern of eggplant purple turning to a lovely brown-green and then to yellow before fading out. The amount of bruising varies with each individual and is impossible to accurately forecast. I've seen some women who immediately go right into the final yellow stage, with just dabs of purple here and there. I've also seen women who bruise purple from their forehead clear down to their nipples, but that's the exception. Your doctor will instruct you when to use warm or cold compresses to assist in relieving both the swelling and bruising.

Generally you can expect to be almost bruise-free by the fourth week after surgery. But don't worry. You won't have to hide for weeks. After about a week, if you're not discharging from an incision line and your eyes are infection-free, you can cover your existing bruises with makeup while they're taking their time to fade. Certain cosmetics cover bruising much more effectively than others, and I'll get into that in detail in the next chapter. *Do not* apply makeup to any incision line before 48 hours after suture removal.

Know that you will be closely monitored by your doctor during a series of post-op checkups, the first being the day following surgery. If you've had your eyes done, some stitches are removed the fourth or fifth day following surgery. Seven to 10 days post-op, your face-lift stitches around the front of your ears are removed. Some stitches may be left in. If so, they're self-dissolving. If you had a forehead (or coronal) lift, the staples or stitches are removed 12 to 14 days after surgery, and the staples or stitches running diagonally behind the ears and up into the hairline are removed 10 to 14 days post-op. Office staff nurses will often remove stitches, staples, casts and so on. They are usually extremely skilled at all of this, and you needn't worry about allowing them to do their job.

You are normally checked again a week later and then for a final time four to six weeks after surgery. Of course, if you have ANY concerns about even the smallest pain, call your doctor that same day. Go in and let him see what you consider to be a problem. If it's a real issue, the doctor will treat it appropriately. If it is just part of your normal healing process, at least you'll get reassured and will be able to relax again.

Incision lines have a distinctive healing process. They are bright pink in color before they fade to an unnoticeable white scar. The incisions that run in front of the ear contour normally remain quite thin. However, the incision that runs behind the ear tends to look wide and ropy at first, almost like gathered fabric. This ropiness eventually flattens out completely and the pinkness disappears.

You may have a small incision line under your chin, most probably just covered with surgical tape. The incision is made if your surgeon feels it is necessary to liposuction out some fat in order to give your face a sleeker line. The tape is usually removed the fourth day post-op; the incision line will flatten out and turn colorless like the others.

THE POSTSURGERY BLUES

The subject of depression following surgery is worth examining. Most offices will mention the possibility of a couple of days of mild depression during the first week after surgery. Some women I've worked with experienced little or no depression, but many people can expect a few really gloomy days. This is a result of postsurgical letdown combined with the physical trauma of the surgery itself, the anesthesia gradually wearing off, physical exhaustion and the shock of seeing yourself so distorted and banged up and generally unpretty.

My attitude is, if you want to cry, go ahead and cry. But don't take it to the extremes that I frequently hear, such as, "I've destroyed myself, I look like a freak," or, "That S.O.B. doctor turned me into a monster!"

If you feel yourself careening into hysteria, stop and regroup. Remind yourself that in all probability no one has destroyed you— almost everyone looks horrible at first. *It will all pass.* And as long as you understand that the depression will pass, too, you can say to yourself, "OK, so I'm depressed. So what? It'll be gone soon."

The key word to your recovery period three weeks after surgery is: *surrender.* Just surrender to it all. If you feel blue, cry a little. If you're exhausted, rest, and don't try to do more than your body can easily tolerate. If you hate the way you're swollen and bruised, realize it will all go away. Just surrender to the situation, to all your anxiety and fatigue. Know that it will all go away. In spite of your worst nightmares, in spite of all your apprehensions, it will all go away. As long as you know this, believe me, you can go through any normal healing process and not feel panicked or victimized.

The first week following surgery you shouldn't be doing much more than resting. There's no need to be completely bed-bound. however. You can walk around the house and even take brief walks if you like, but for the most part, take it easy. If you go for a walk, be sure to wear a large brimmed hat. You don't want any sun on your face, especially on the incision lines. The sun can darken your bruises and incision lines permanently, so keep your face shaded, and once your doctor give his OK, you can apply sunscreen to your scars for the first year post-surgery.

Do not lift anything heavy and do not attempt any housework or physically stressful activity. You have many permanent stitches under your skin in muscles and other areas, in addition to the stitches you can see externally. The last thing you want to do is pull them and perhaps create some bleeding or an unnecessary problem. So be smart and don't overdo it. Just relax as much as possible, move around a little, and rest.

You'll be sent home with antibiotics and steroids. It's very important that you complete the full course of both medications. After the first week, if you are completely off your pain medication and feeling more mobile, you can begin to drive again. Be careful not to turn and twist your neck too much during this period. Try to rotate your entire torso along with your head when looking left and right. By the end of the second week, it's helpful to stand under the shower and let the warm water run onto your neck while you gently rotate your head from side to side. You need to be moving your neck normally by the third week after the operation. You don't want the muscles to atrophy.

For those of you who love your exercise and hiking and tennis, forget it for four to six weeks following surgery. Your doctor will tell you exactly when it's safe to return to specific routines. For instance, no aerobics until six weeks post-op. If you return to exercising too soon, your swelling will continue much longer than normal, and you could run the risk of unnecessary complications. It's smarter to take it easy for a few weeks and have a face that's well and problem-free forever.

You'll be able to brush your teeth gently, but stay on soft foods and avoid heavy chewing and excessive talking for about a week. You'll be using Polysporin Ointment to clean the sutures. *Do not* put alcohol, vaseline or other ointments and creams on the incision lines unless instructed to by your doctor. Some itching of healing wounds is to be expected; *do not scratch them!*

The anesthetics and pain medications tend to produce constipation, so it's wise to eat high-fiber foods or take stool softeners during recovery. You mustn't put any strain on your incision lines, and that includes stress on the entire body created by "bearing down" on the toilet if you're constipated. If you experience diarrhea call your doctor, as it may be due to medication such as an antibiotic.

NUMBNESS AND OTHER NORMAL REACTIONS

Another adjustment you should be prepared for during recovery is temporary numbness. After a face-lift, the cheek area in front of your ears will be numb for about eight months to one year. As always, there will be exceptions, and you may normalize much faster than most people. The sides of the neck also usually remain numb and feel tight for up to a year. Most women describe their postsurgical neck as similar to wearing a vise. *Don't worry!* As the swelling leaves the neck area, that uncomfortably "confined" sensation will disappear. However, the tight feeling will not vanish completely until as much as a year after surgery. Look at it this way: You wanted a nice, new, taut neck. And you got it! There is a vertical row of permanent stitches beneath your skin on either side of your neck, ensuring it stays just the way you like it for the next few years. That's why it feels so tight. Like everything else, it will eventually soften up and feel perfectly normal again. Because your face is partially numb following surgery, you'll have no way of assessing temperature damage, so *do not put ice directly on the skin*, and *do not put heating pads on the skin.*

If you've had a coronal forehead-lift, you will wake up from surgery feeling like you're wearing a bathing cap that's a couple of sizes too small. This particular procedure may be terribly uncomfortable for people who suffer from migraines. The tight-cap feeling, as well as the numbness on the scalp, could last 8 to 12 weeks. You must be especially careful during this period not to accidentally burn yourself with hot hair dryers, curling irons or electric rollers. It will be impossible to judge what's too hot until your normal feeling returns. The safest policy until then is to use all hair appliances on medium or low settings.

As for numbness following eye surgery, the eye area usually begins to feel normal again three to six weeks after the operation.

All of the numbness I've listed is similar to the Novocaine sensation you experience at the dentist. Just transpose that feeling to the specific areas where you'll be having your surgery, and you'll know exactly what to expect until the numbness normalizes. Periods of tingling and small shooting pains can also occur, but it's all part of your normal healing process.

The only areas that actually hurt following a face-lift seem to be the incision lines at the ears. Most people have real soreness and tenderness there for about five weeks. This makes it rather difficult to sleep on your side during that period. You will be instructed by your doctor to sleep propped up for a specific time, depending on what surgery you had. After you're through your propped-up period, try to invent a comfortable sleeping device to spare yourself the sore-ear syndrome. Some people sleep with their head and temple balanced on the arm of one of those bed backrests.

Remember to take your pain and sleeping medications if you need them. Your doctor will know your medical history, and if you have any problems with drug dependency before your surgery your medication will be prescribed accordingly. You don't need to be a martyr, nor should you feel intimidated by your recovery medication. It's there to help you get through any uncomfortable moments. Also, keep in mind that you heal faster when you're more relaxed, so a good night's sleep is important.

If you've had eye surgery, you can expect to have slightly out-of-focus vision for a few weeks post-op. This is because the eyeball itself swells up a little, but like everything else, the condition is only temporary.

Your skin usually goes through a change right after surgery. People who never had pimples can suddenly break out. Your skin can become quite dry and flaky or turn excessively oily. Ignore it. It's a combination of trauma and the anesthesia being eliminated from the system, and it will pass in three to four weeks.

The anesthesia also does something dismal to your hair, but only temporarily. In essence, your hair "commits suicide" for about three months after surgery. It becomes limp and loses its shine, and in many cases will even thin out a little. *Do not panic!* The good news is that when it finally comes back in, it's thicker and fuller than ever, as is often common during pregnancy. Eight out of 10 women I've worked with have been relieved and thrilled to eventually have a better head of hair than they did prior to surgery.

Be sure to check with your doctor before coloring your hair after surgery. Generally you must wait until four weeks post-op before coloring. However, everybody's different and your doctor may want you to wait longer. Ask him specifically about coloring, perming, chemical straightening and any other treatment you use.

It is also common for many people to experience some temporary memory loss combined with what I refer to as "dumbs disease." You know, that fuzzy state where you just can't seem to "get it together." *Relax—you're not going crazy!* You're just a little shocked and exhausted. Your thinking process will be clear and normal in two or three weeks.

The exhaustion following your surgery can vary from mild to quite extreme. Most people feel as if they've been hit by a truck for the first couple of weeks. Your energy level will slowly and surely climb back up, but don't expect that to happen in any consistent upswing. For the first couple of weeks, as mentioned, you can be seriously fatigued. Then you'll feel absolutely wonderful for a day, and perhaps lousy for the next two. Great for three days straight…tired the fourth. Your energy level usually will improve in this up-and-down pattern until the fourth week. By then you should be looking and feeling quite well, and your energy will continue to rise steadily until the eighth week, when it will most likely be back to normal.

Most people don't feel peppy enough to resume any sexual activity for a few weeks. After, and only after all of your sutures have been removed (personally, I'd wait at least a full week after), you can *gently* resume your sexual activities. Remember, no stress or strain on your face or any incision lines, so forget wild sex and swinging from chandeliers for another several weeks.

Always remember, the keyword for your recovery period is *surrender.* If you're exhausted, rest. If you're depressed, let yourself be sad for an instant. Just don't overdo anything and delay your healing process. *And above all, know that it will all go away in just a little while. Soon you will feel like your old self again, and you will love the way you look!*

CHAPTER SIX

Corrective Makeup After Surgery and Basic Makeup Tricks

• • •

You can start to wear cosmetics on your face to cover your bruises about a week after surgery, but don't put any makeup over your incision lines until a minimum of 48 hours after the sutures have been removed. If your incision lines are not completely healed and dry 48 hours following suture removal, consult your doctor about when it would be safe for you to use cosmetics on the area.

Liquid makeups are completely useless in covering postsurgical bruising. Two of the best products available for this three-to-four week period are Physicians Formula Velvet Film or Max Factor Pan Stick. Both products are cream-based foundations that will provide the coverage you'll need to camouflage the initial discoloration. Actually, any cream-based foundation will work as long as it's not too oily.

You should purchase the foundation just prior to surgery. Ask to see the testers similar to your skin tone, and match the color closest to the skin at the base of your throat area. Your face and neck could be so multicolored after surgery that you'll want your coverage to match your body. Apply sample strips of makeup to the throat and upper chest area, then take a mirror and walk outside into the daylight to determine your closest color match. If you're extremely fair and your color is an ivory tone, you'll probably have to go slightly darker with the color foundation in order to provide coverage. Anything paler than the beige tones doesn't really give adequate coverage for those first three weeks of bruising.

The key to applying foundation is to use only the minimum amount of makeup necessary to even out the discoloration. *The only mistake you can make when applying cosmetics is to use too much.* First, put on a little moisturizer and then gently apply the foundation with a dry foam-rubber wedge sponge over the entire face and neck area, including the eyelids and under eyes. Where your bruises are more pronounced, gently pat some additional foundation over the area and *stop* the instant the color has evened out. Those deep, eggplant-purple bruises are very difficult to cover, and you may need to pat a product called Dermablend over them. Dermablend is a very thick, dry cream used for difficult skin discolorations; it can be purchased in most department stores. Other products that will cover deep purple bruises include Clinique Continuous Coverage, Prescriptives Camouflage Creme, Lydia O'Leary Cover Mark or Linda Seidel's Natural Cover. Again, the lighter the coverage you can get away with, the better you'll look.

Once the foundation color looks as even as possible, dust the face and neck with the barest amount of loose translucent powder. The powder must be applied with a soft brush. If you apply it with a powder puff or with a cotton ball, it will look too heavy. To ensure the minimum amount, you'll want to make certain that you blow the powder off the brush before applying. As your bruising begins to disappear, you'll be using less foundation each day and then finally returning to your usual brand of makeup. Many women use a liquid foundation, which looks particularly good when combined with a drop of moisturizer. Just put a pea-sized drop of foundation in the palm of your hand, add an equal drop of moisturizer and mix them together with a cotton swab. Using the swab, dot the entire face with the makeup and blend it out evenly with a foam sponge. This will give a sheer, natural look to your skin.

If you're only slightly bruised, you may actually be able to use your own brand of liquid makeup by the second week after surgery, combined with a matching color cream foundation on the discolored areas only. The cream makeup can be applied right over the liquid foundation and, as always, use the lightest touch while blending the edges of the cream makeup out with the sponge. You'll want to achieve a look where the cream makeup areas just seem to disappear into the sheer liquid foundation. It's a bit tricky, but you can do it with a little practice and a featherweight dabbing technique of blending the two areas together. As long as you have any bruises remaining on your face, it's best to continue to dust a few grains of powder over the area to prevent the discoloration from bleeding through the makeup.

Once you've powdered your face, it's best to use a powder blush on the cheeks. Never try to apply a cream blush over powdered cheeks—it just won't go on smoothly. If you love your cream blush, use it over a cream foundation, powdering last.

The following rule for applying blush applies to everyone, regardless of the shape of your face. Starting from the center of the apple of your cheek when you smile, run your blush back across your cheek, aiming for the big hole in your ear. This will probably place the color lower than you normally apply it. However, this is the correct position for blush. It will slim down your cheeks, make your cheekbones appear higher and place everything in correct proportion. When the blush is placed too high on the cheekbone the face can appear too long. Aim for the big hole in your ear, and you'll never go wrong. Also, dust a little blush across the bottom of the chin, on the temples and on the tip of the nose so that your color is evenly distributed over the face. Remember to blend these areas out with your foam sponge.

Apply the powder blush with a soft brush, using short dabbing strokes rather than long continuous strokes. The dabbing application blends the color out more evenly. Try to stay in natural colors of rose, peach or coral. Blush shades that tend toward brown and grayish tones usually have an aging effect on the faces of people older than the mid-twenties—and who needs that after going through all this surgery!

One of the biggest mistakes most women make after a face-lift is to apply too much makeup. Many women are accustomed to trying to correct specific problems, such as sagging eyelids and droopy cheeks, with an overkill makeup. But guess what? You've just gone through surgery to correct what you disliked, and you don't have to follow your old makeup habits anymore! When applying any makeup to your face, always remember one thing: *Less is better.* Being overly made-up not only looks terrible, it also ages the face.

Everything you put on your face should be the minimum amount of product. Always blow your powder, blush or eye makeup off the brush before applying it to your face so you'll never have to worry about looking too highly colored.

It doesn't really matter what brand of product you choose. Some of the products I use are from the drug store, others are more expensive name brands that I purchased because the color appealed to me. The entire secret to using makeup lies in the colors you choose, where you place those colors on your bone structure and how you blend it all in.

Choose a foundation that is as close as possible to the color of your neck. Nothing looks worse than a color difference between the face and body, so always match your foundation to the neck rather than the skin tone on your face. As mentioned before, apply it with a drop of moisturizer to give your skin a sheer appearance.

After all your bruising has disappeared, you may want to dust a few grains of powder only on your cheeks, as a primer for a powder blush. The skin seems to look younger and more natural without powder but again, it's a matter of personal taste.

When applying your lipstick, do not outline your lips with a pencil that's a darker color than the lipstick itself. Apart from looking terribly hard, it looks very sixties and unnatural and will immediately age you. Choose a lip pencil color that's one shade lighter than your lipstick. It will accomplish the "finished" look you want on your mouth without being obvious.

Eye makeup should also remain simple. Be sure to put a drop of foundation on your eyelids before applying any eye shadow. Your eye makeup will stay on all day when it has a base to adhere to. Use muted colors, whether they're natural earth tones, soft khakis or quiet plums and violets. Bright colors draw too much attention to the makeup itself and are very difficult to wear unless you're a twenty-year-old cover girl.

What follows is a fast and beautiful three-step eye makeup routine that's virtually fail-safe:

1. Cover the entire eyelid from lashes straight up into the eyebrow with any pale muted color, such as peach, pale brown or soft violet. Use your foam sponge with a drop of foundation on it, and pat over the entire area to blend out the color and eliminate any color edges. The purpose of applying a pale color over the entire lid area is to flatten back the brow bone and open up the eye

area even larger. Do not apply white eyeshadow to the brow bone, as it will instantly close down the look of the eye.

2. Line your eye with a darker color: Dark brown if your lid is covered in an earth tone, navy blue if your lid is covered in a pale violet or pink tone. Throw out your black eyeliner; it will instantly age the appearance of your face. Some women love the look of lining the eyes in powder eyeshadow. It gives a very soft, smoky look and is incredibly easy and quick. Apply the darker eye shadow as an eyeliner with a small, soft, diagonal brush. The only thing you'll need to remember when lining with powder eye shadow is to blow it off the brush like mad before applying, so the powder doesn't crumble down your face and create a mess. Line the top lid from inside corner to outside corner. What's nice about lining in powder is that you don't need to be precise. Just throw it on as wide as you like, and smudge it out with your finger to create the appearance of a darker area near your lashes, floating up into the paler color on the lid. When lining under the eye, you must keep the line thin and narrow. In fact, use a smaller regular eyeliner brush for under the eye and only line from the outside corner into the center of the eye. Again, take the sponge with your foundation on it and dab at this under-eye line so it always seems pale and soft. Don't run the eyeliner clear across the bottom lid, as it will draw your eyes too close together. Let it disappear at the center of the eye. If you prefer a harder edge eye makeup, then line with a dark brown or navy pencil, cake or liquid makeup, but use a light touch with anything you use.

3. Mascara upper and lower lashes with black mascara, even if you're a blonde. I always wipe the wand off with Kleenex before applying because I dislike the look of globby mascara.

Eyebrows should be kept as natural as possible. Using the same type of small, soft, diagonal brush you used to line your lids, fill in your brows with a dark brown powder eyeshadow, not an eyebrow pencil. The result will be much more real. If you make your eyebrows darker than your hair color, your face will look much younger and more expressive. A great color both for eyebrows and as a dark brown eyeliner is a powder eyeshadow by Lancôme called Lezard. It's a very rich brown that looks good on almost everyone. As always, blow it off the brush before applying, and use a light touch.

For evening makeup, use the same color tones everywhere, but you can apply everything slightly heavier for a more dramatic effect. Another good evening look is to add a step to the above routine and run a black eye pencil across the inside of your lower eyelid. Make sure the lead in the pencil is very soft for easy and painless application. Almay makes a great black eye pencil that slides right on. The effect of this black pencil does tend to make the eye seem a little smaller, but it can be a very beautiful and theatrical addition for a dressy evening.

The purpose of makeup is to make your face seem even and beautiful. Makeup should be easy and quick and fun. The last thing you want to do is to destroy the success of your wonderful new surgery with old makeup habits.

As long as you remember that *less is best*, you'll always look appealing.

EXAMPLE OF DAYTIME EYE (LEFT, BELOW)

① *Cover entire lid with soft, neutral color earthtone eye shadow.*

② *Line eyes with darker earthtone color eyeshadow. Remember to keep the bottom eyeliner very thin and not beyond the center of the eye.*

③ *Blush is brushed on from the center of the apple of the cheek to the opening of the ear.*

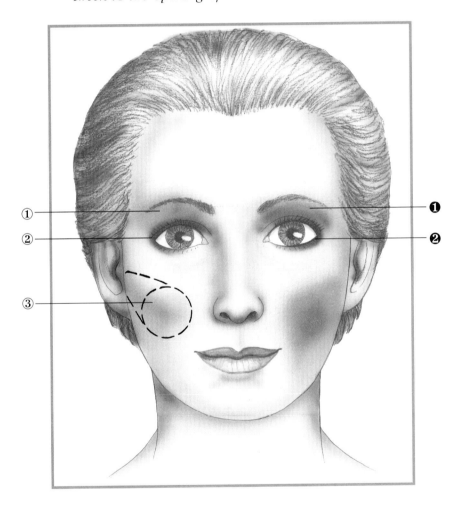

EXAMPLE OF EVENING EYE (RIGHT, ABOVE)

❶ *Eyeshadow tones can be applied slightly darker for evening wear.*

❷ *A soft black eye pencil on the bottom lid can give some added glamour.*

Part Two: Other Surgeries

CHAPTER SEVEN

Eyelid Surgery

• • •

APPROXIMATE COST:

Upper lids: $2,700–$3,500

Lower lids: $2,700–$3,500

There may be additional charges for surgical facilities and anesthesia. Be sure to request this information.

APPROXIMATE TIME UNTIL COMPLETELY HEALED:

Five to eight weeks.

PRESURGICAL INSTRUCTIONS

- You will be given blood and lab tests approximately two weeks before surgery. Take no aspirin or aspirin-containing products for two weeks prior to your surgery and one week after (see list of medications to avoid). They can cause bleeding and bruising. You may take Tylenol.

- Avoid sunbathing the face for two weeks prior to surgery.

- If you take medication daily, notify your doctor. Also inform him if you develop an illness, cold or any skin infections about the face and neck within a week of your surgery.

- If you're a smoker, you should clearly understand that nicotine can impair and delay healing. Most offices will suggest quitting a week to 10 days before surgery, and a week post-op. If it were me, I'd stop smoking a minimum of three weeks prior to surgery and not touch a cigarette for a full month post-op. Who needs to be left with scars worse than normal as well as other complications as a result of smoking through the pre- and post-surgical period?

THE DAY BEFORE SURGERY

- Do not eat or drink anything after midnight.

- The night before surgery, shower and shampoo your hair and cleanse your face.

THE DAY OF SURGERY

- You may rinse and brush your teeth, but do *not eat or drink anything.* Some offices may ask you to take pills with a small amount of water the day of surgery.

- Wear no makeup and remove contact lenses and dentures for surgery. *Do not put any moisturizer on your eyes or face.*

- Do not bring any jewelry or valuables. Wear a robe, housecoat or warmup suit that buttons or zips in the front, and wear flat shoes. *No tight-fitting clothes.*

- *Someone must drive you home and stay with you the first night.*

- Postoperative instructions regarding activity, medications and office visits will be given to you following your surgery.

THE SURGERY

Upper eyelid surgery takes approximately one hour. Lower eyelid surgery also runs about an hour. Add an additional half hour for preparation and anesthesia. There are normally four people in the operating room with you: the surgeon, the anesthesiologist, and two surgical nurses.

You will be given a general anesthetic intravenously. An I.V. antibiotic will also be administered.

UPPER EYELIDS

First, locations are marked for the incision line on the upper eyelid. This may be done while the patient is in a seated position to correspond to how you will see yourself in a standing position. (Marking the incision lines in a reclined posture would produce a different result.)

Excess skin is removed with special care to place the incision in the normal fold of the upper eyelid and also to avoid removing eyebrow skin. It's important that the incision allow at least 1-1/2 centimeters between the fold of the eyelid and the eyebrow. Otherwise the eyelid won't blend into the brow and the end result would be very unacceptable.

After opening the eyelid skin and removing the excess, the muscle of the upper eyelid is opened, and the fat that tends to cause the bulging is removed. Most people are particularly aware of the fat in the middle corner of the eyelid. This is usually removed with an electric cautery, which coagulates the blood vessels and stops the bleeding. The wound is then closed with skin stitches.

LOWER EYELIDS

Most surgeons make an incision just under the lash margin to remove the excess fat and, to a minimal degree, the excess skin. The incision is then closed with stitches. It's becoming increasingly popular to remove the fat through an incision on the inside of the eyelid, leaving no scar on the face. However, this procedure must be combined with the incision just under the lashes if excess skin is to be removed.

POSTSURGICAL INSTRUCTIONS

1. Apply ice compresses to eyes almost constantly during the waking hours for the first 24 hours after surgery. Thereafter they may be used as you need them to relieve itching or discomfort. Use four-by-four-inch gauze pads soaked in ice water and wrung out damp. *Do not put ice* directly on skin. *Do not use eye drops* unless instructed to do so.

2. Continue your antibiotics until your doctor instructs you to stop.

3. Swelling and discoloration are expected and will begin to subside about three days after surgery. You may take a stool softener if you are constipated.

4. For comfort, warm compresses may be used five days following surgery and thereafter.

5. Limit yourself to light activities for one week. Sleep with head elevated.

6. Avoid straining, vigorous exercise, or the head-down position, all of which may cause excessive pressure in the eyes and may encourage unnecessary swelling or bleeding.

7. Consider discomfort as an indication that you have been too active—rest and apply cold compresses. Only after that should you consider taking pain medication stronger than acetaminophen (Tylenol).

8. If you experience dryness or scratchiness of the eyes, use artificial tears such as HypoTears, Tears Naturale or Lacrilube. These may be used as much as you desire.

9. Wear sunglasses when exposed to sun rays to protect eyelids for four to six weeks.

10. You may wash your face and shampoo your hair. Thoroughly rinse after washing to remove any soap or shampoo residues.

11. Makeup may be used over intact skin, but do not apply it to wounds with sutures or to incision lines before 48 hours after suture removal.

12. Make an appointment to return for suture removal approximately five days after surgery.

THE RECOVERY PERIOD

You'll have two lovely shiners following your surgery, particularly if you've had the lower eyelids done too. The bruises are usually a deep purple color before turning brown, green, yellow and then fading to normal. The purple bruises under the eyes are always the most stubborn and can linger for up to four or five weeks post-op, and sometimes longer. The good news is that *they will eventually completely disappear,* and you can cover them with makeup (Dermablend, Prescriptives Camouflage Creme, Cover Mark, Natural Cover or Clinique Continuous Coverage) until they're gone. Be sure that you don't apply any makeup to wounds with sutures. Medically, it's reasonably safe to apply some makeup to the incision lines 48 hours after suture removal, but I wouldn't advise using makeup around incision lines for a good week post-op unless it is absolutely necessary.

Almost all incision lines "raise up" and become quite pink before they flatten out; it's part of the normal healing process. The incision lines also tend to look lumpy before they flatten, and they can even develop small cysts that will easily be removed by your doctor.

You will experience a tight-eye sensation for a good three to four weeks. Don't worry—as your swelling begins to subside, the tight feeling will ease up and finally return to normal.

Heavy eye tearing can occur one to three weeks post-op. Also, don't be surprised if your vision seems soft and slightly out of focus for three or four weeks; the actual eyeball swells slightly as a result of the surgery in the area. Like everything else, it all normalizes with time.

Expect a slight clear mucous buildup around the lids following surgery. This occurs because the swelling has temporarily closed the tear duct. Artificial tears will help clear the eyes until the problem corrects itself.

You mustn't even attempt to wear contact lenses until you have your doctor's OK. The lenses won't fit a swollen eyeball, and they're impossible to remove if you put them in during the swollen period.

Any eye exercises should be done only at your doctor's request. This includes no reading for 48 hours. Television is okay after 24 hours.

PROBLEM SIGNS

Any type of serious pain should be reported to your doctor immediately. Any heavy oozing from incision lines or any excess pus should be considered abnormal and reported to your doctor. Bleeding in the area or an eye that's glued shut from excessive amounts of secreted matter are problems your doctor needs to know about as soon as the symptom occurs. Allergic symptoms such as excessive redness and itching are problems. You could be allergic to the Polysporin or other medication.

MAKEUP TRICKS

Once you've been told by your doctor that it's safe to apply eye makeup—usually 48 hours after suture removal—run a little cream foundation over the entire lid and undereye area. The bruises that are very purple and dark will bleed through the foundation and appear to be a deep grey color. Take the smallest amount of Dermablend, Clinique Continuous Coverage, Prescriptives Camouflage Creme, Cover Mark or Natural Cover in your appropriate color, and lightly dab it on right over the cream foundation. The instant the bruise is covered, *stop applying makeup*. It's important that any makeup you use match the color of the cream foundation you're using. If it's too pale, you'll end up looking ghoulish and pasty.

Once you've evened out your skin tone, you can apply your usual eye makeup. However, *do not* use eyelash curlers or eyelash tints until the end of the eighth week post-op. It's also a good idea to avoid the mauve, plum and blue tones of eye shadow color during your bruised period of recovery. These colors tend to make your bruising look worse even through camouflage makeup. Stay in the earth tones until your bruising has disappeared.

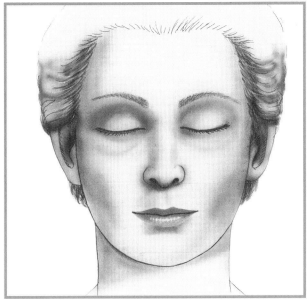

Prior to surgery, drooping upper eyelids, loose lower eyelids and fat pads are often the main complaints.

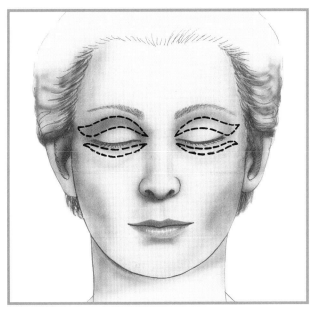

Incision lines are placed in the normal fold of the upper eyelid and just under the lash margin of the lower lid.

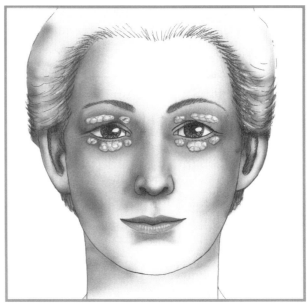

Underlying areas of fat and excess skin will be removed from the area.

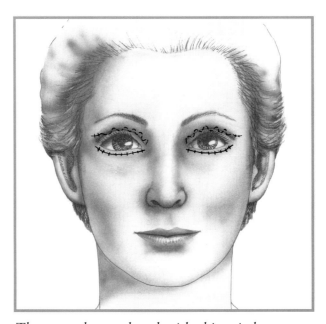

The wounds are closed with skin stitches.

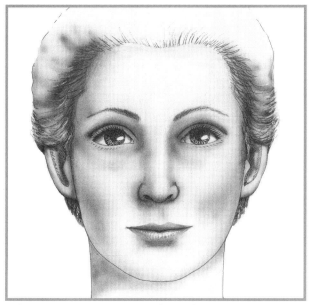

The postoperative eye is free of sagging upper lids and shows a firm and even area under the eye.

CHAPTER EIGHT

Rhinoplasty

(NASAL SURGERY)

• • •

APPROXIMATE COST: $2,800–$6,800

There may be additional charges for surgical facilities and anesthesia. Be sure to request this information.

APPROXIMATE TIME UNTIL COMPLETELY HEALED:

Nine months to one year.

BEFORE YOU SET A DATE FOR SURGERY

It's imperative that you meet with your doctor at least twice prior to nasal surgery so you can both be absolutely clear and in agreement over the desired look of your new nose. There's nothing worse than a "surprise nose" sitting in the middle of your face for the rest of your life, so get very specific about what you want. The very best way to communicate your preferences is to bring your doctor pictures from fashion magazines showing examples of the size and shape of the nose you have in mind. Any decisions regarding the shape of your new nose should take into account the shape of your chin. Your new profile must achieve a beautiful balance between the nose and chin. If the chin is receding, an implant often is appropriate to create the correct facial symmetry.

The concept of rhinoplasty is to refine, realign and reposition the nasal tissues. This is accomplished by rearranging cartilage and bone to alter the shape of the nose. Reducing the general size of the nose, removing a nasal hump, reshaping the tip or correcting an unattractive angle between the nose and the upper lip, all can be achieved in a single operation. Tissue often must be added to improve the silhouette of the nose; cartilage is obtained from the septums or the external ear for this purpose.

PRESURGICAL INSTRUCTIONS

- If you take medication daily, notify your doctor. You will be given blood and lab tests approximately two weeks prior to surgery. Take no aspirin or aspirin-containing products for two weeks prior to and one week after your surgery. Aspirin can cause bleeding and bruising. You may take acetaminophen (Tylenol).

- Avoid sunbathing the face for two weeks prior to surgery.

- If you develop a cold or other illness within a week of your surgery, or if you develop any skin infections about the face and neck, notify your doctor.

- If you're a smoker you should clearly understand that nicotine can impair and delay healing. Most offices will suggest quitting a week to 10 days before surgery, a week post-op. If it were me, I'd stop smoking a minimum of three weeks prior to surgery and not touch a cigarette for a full month post-op. Who needs to be left with scars worse than normal and other complications as a result of smoking through the pre- and postsurgical period?

THE DAY BEFORE SURGERY

- Do not eat or drink anything after midnight. Some offices may ask you to take pills with a small amount of water the day of surgery.

- The night before or the morning of surgery, shower and shampoo your hair.

THE DAY OF SURGERY

- Rinse and brush your teeth but *do not eat or drink anything.* Wear no makeup and remove contact lenses. Do not apply moisturizer on your eyelids or facial skin.

- Wear a robe, housecoat or warmup suit that buttons or zips in the front, and wear flat shoes. *No tight-fitting clothes.*

- *Someone must drive you home on the day of your surgery.*

- Postoperative instructions regarding dressings, activity, medications, suture removal and office visits will be given following your surgery.

THE SURGERY

The surgery takes approximately an hour and a half to two hours. Add an additional half hour for preparation and anesthesia. You will be given antibiotics to combat potential infections. There are normally four people in the operating room with you: the surgeon, the anesthesiologist and two surgical nurses. You will be given a general anesthetic intravenously. An I.V. antibiotic will also be administered.

The entire procedure is performed from inside the nose. Surgery usually begins with work on the septums. Not everyone has septum work, but it's rather common because many people require breathing corrections.

Incisions are made on either side of the nose inside the vestibule (nostril). The tissue, cartilage, fat and skin are "freed-up" (separated) from the overlying bone. Work on the profile includes rasping (filing) the hump down or actually removing it with a fine saw or a chisel. The nasal bones are then cut at their base running vertically at either side of the nose, and are moved inward to form a narrower bridge. If the nasal tip needs elevating, the septum will be trimmed through the incisions in the nostrils. Other tip work, such as reshaping cartilage and definition of the nasal tip, also is performed via these incisions. Twelve to 15 ministitches are taken to close up the incisions inside the nostrils. They are absorbable and will dissolve on their own. Occasionally the doctor may elect to combine the nostril incisions with an incision across the column of the nose. This is the fleshy part between the nostrils. This operation is called open rhinoplasty, and it results in a fine, usually inconspicuous scar in this area.

If the base of the nose is too wide, wedges of the skin are removed and the nostrils are brought closer to the columella (the column between the nostrils) to produce a narrower nose. Tiny scars will remain where the sutures were placed, but they can be camouflaged with makeup after the nose has healed.

Packing is usually inserted in the nostrils to protect the septum for three to five days, and a tape-and-plastic splint or a plaster overlay is applied to adhere the tissue and support the new shape of the bone for about a week.

An alternative surgical procedure for lifting the nose is to make incision lines at the base of the column separating the nostrils and around the base and outside curve of the nostrils, and then lift the entire nose upward. Some doctors approve of this technique, but it will leave you with a visible scar under the tip of your nose.

NASAL IMPLANTS

Implants often are placed in the nose to correct the look of a broad, flat nose or the lack of a bridge. They are also used in reconstruction following accidents. The implant is inserted through an incision inside the nostril.

Synthetic implants are tolerated very well in Asians and African Americans, but Caucasians seem to have problems with them, and the removal rate is as high as 60 percent. Caucasians should opt for cartilage implants in the nose. Cartilage implants are well tolerated by all races.

POSTSURGICAL INSTRUCTIONS

1. Rest at home and limit yourself to light activities for one week.

2. Continue your antibiotics until your doctor instructs you to stop.

3. Frequently change the "moustache dressing"—the gauze under your nostrils—to catch any light bleeding from the nose. You may need to change it four or five times an hour for the first two to three hours after surgery. Then, as the bleeding diminishes, the dressing will probably require changing one to two times an hour until the morning.

4. Vigorous sports or exercises that cause straining should be curtailed for six weeks following surgery. You may gently swim in

a swimming pool after a time to be determined by your doctor. *No diving* for two months.

5. Sleep and rest with head comfortably elevated.

6. Do not blow your nose until advised, and then do so gently, one nostril at a time.

7. If you wear glasses you will be shown how to tape them up off the bridge of your nose for approximately six weeks.

8. Do not sunbathe or burn the nose for six weeks after surgery.

9. If you sneeze, open your mouth widely.

10. If you have nasal packing, it may be removed three to five days after the operation. Often it will fall out (partially or fully) prior to that time. Gentle removal or cutting the protruding portion with scissors is appropriate. If the packing is still in your nose on your return visit, the doctor or nurse will remove it for you.

11. The splint should remain dry. It will be removed on your return at five to seven days after the operation.

THE RECOVERY PERIOD

Be prepared to be annoyed by the packing in your nose. It's uncomfortable, and although it's a tube-packing with a tiny hole in the center for air, you'll end up having to breathe through your mouth until the packing is removed. One nice improvement is that today's tube packing is coated and slips out of the nose quite painlessly.

Unlike the painless face-lift, any work on the nose will leave you quite uncomfortable, tender and sore for a good week to 10 days. The nose will remain very tender to the touch—sensitive even to the weight of a washcloth—for about six weeks post-op. But don't worry, it never gets really terrible, and it all passes with time.

You'll probably wake up with a couple of black eyes and some more bruising on the nose. The bruising usually is gone in 10 to 14 days.

You'll be swollen, of course. You really won't be able to judge your new nose for the first four months after surgery. That initial swelling makes it look fatter and wider than you perhaps imagined, but by the fifth month, you'll like what you see. However, you should know that it takes a full nine months to a year for all of the swelling to disappear following rhinoplasty.

Your nose will be stuffy for about two or three weeks following surgery. Be prepared for a constant dry throat, because you'll be breathing through your mouth a lot during this period. Throat lozenges are very helpful, and if your doctor says it's OK, an antihistamine at night could help open up your breathing passages.

Take it very easy for the first weeks following surgery—rest and do only very light activities. Absolutely no exercising or heavy physical activities, not even bending, for six to eight weeks. You don't want to do anything that will raise blood pressure or create nose bleeding.

You'll be able to return to work a week to 10 days following surgery. You'll be slightly tired, swollen and bruised, but you can resume your work routine as long as it's not overly physical.

Some years ago an eight-year-old child accidentally broke my nose. The break was camouflaged with a cartilage implant, and the septum was realigned. I was surprised to experience a kind of shaky and fragile recovery from nasal surgery. Apparently most people feel a bit more vulnerable following rhinoplasty than after a full face-lift. The nose is an extremely sensitive area. But even at its worst, rhinoplasty is never an unbearable experience. It's uncomfortable and fatiguing and tender for a while, and then it all passes and you're fine again.

One large "possible catch" you should prepare yourself for is that 15 to 30 percent of all nasal surgery will require a second touch-up surgery. This is because the surgeon cannot judge how the body will respond to bone rasping (filing) and cutting. The minute a bone is rasped or cut, it thickens while healing. The surgeon must guess how much to remove knowing the bone will thicken. Sometimes he guesses perfectly, but often, the bone will appear slightly larger than desired due to final thickening, and the surgeon will need to go back in nine months to a year post-surgery and remove more bone by further rasping.

Granted, this possibility is a major snag, but it's really not your doctor's fault. He couldn't accurately know how much thickening your body would produce. With luck, you won't need a touch-up surgery, but if you do, know the problem can almost always be fixed.

PROBLEM SIGNS

A small amount of bloody oozing or discharge from the nose is normal. However, any significant bleeding is a problem that requires an immediate call to your doctor. Sometimes the packing needs to be changed, or perhaps it's another type of problem. The rule to remember is, if your nose is bleeding, call your doctor at once.

MAKEUP TRICKS

Once the splint and packing have been removed you can cover the bruises around the eyes and nose with Dermablend, Clinique Continuous Coverage, Prescriptives Camouflage Creme, Cover Mark or Natural Cover sparingly dabbed over the bruised areas and carefully blended out into your normal foundation. *Do not rub* the nose for at least six months following surgery. No rubbing of cosmetics, creams or cosmetic removers. Just gently dab everything on and off.

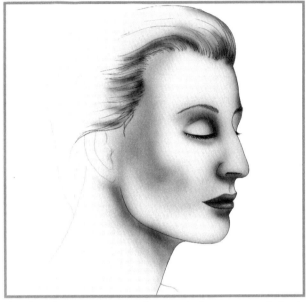

Reshaping your nose is a strictly personal deci-sion as an elective procedure. Be sure to bring pictures of the new nose you'd like as a proto-type for your doctor to study.

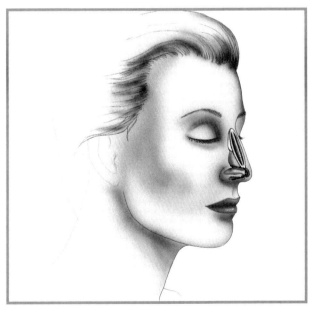

Incisions are made on either side of the nose inside the vestibule. The tissue, cartilage, fat and skin are separated from the bone.

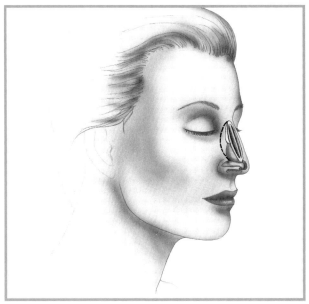

Profile work includes rasping or sawing the hump. The nasal bones are cut at the base on either side of the nose and moved inward to create a narrower bridge.

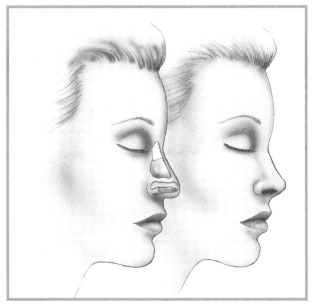

If the nasal tip needs elevating, the septum is trimmed through the incisions in the nostrils.

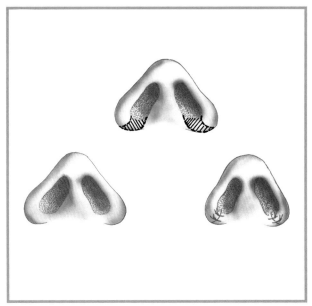

If the base of the nose is too wide, wedges of the skin are removed and the nostrils are brought in closer to the column between the nostrils.

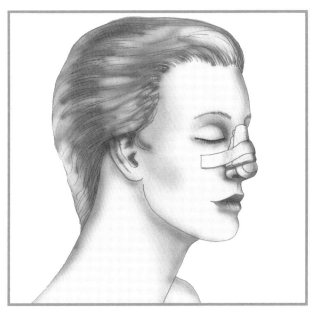

Packing is inserted in the nostrils, and a splint is applied to adhere the tissues and support the new shape of the bone for about a week.

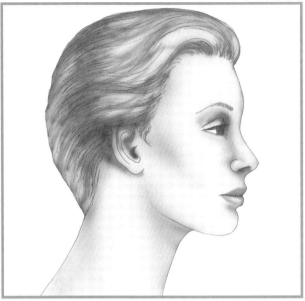

The postoperative nose: smaller and straighter, with a narrower bridge and a refined and elevated tip.

CHAPTER NINE

Brow- and Coronal-Lifts

• • •

APPROXIMATE COST:

Brow-Lift: $1,800

Brow-Pexy: $1,800

Coronal-Lift: $3,000

There may be additional charges for surgical facilities and anesthesia. Be sure to request this information.

APPROXIMATE TIME UNTIL COMPLETELY HEALED:

8 to 12 weeks.

PRESURGICAL INSTRUCTIONS

- You will be given blood and lab tests within two weeks prior to your surgery.

- Take no aspirin or aspirin-containing products (see list of medications to avoid) for two weeks prior to your surgery and one week after. They can cause bleeding and bruising. You may take Tylenol.

- Avoid sunbathing the face for two weeks prior to surgery.

- If you take medication daily, notify your doctor. Also tell him if you develop any illness, a cold or any skin infections about the face and neck within a week of your surgery.

- If you're a smoker, you should clearly understand that nicotine can impair and delay healing. Most offices will suggest quitting a week to 10 days before surgery, a week post-op. If it were me, I'd stop smoking a minimum of three weeks prior to surgery, and not touch a cigarette for a full month post-op. Who needs to be left with scars worse than normal and other complications as a result of smoking through the pre- and postsurgical period?

THE DAY BEFORE SURGERY

Do not eat or drink anything after midnight. The night before surgery, shower and shampoo your hair and cleanse your face. Some offices may ask you to take pills with a small amount of water the day of surgery.

THE DAY OF SURGERY

- You may rinse and brush your teeth, but *do not eat or drink anything* (except your pills, if you were instructed to swallow them the morning of the surgery with the tiniest sip of water).
- Wear no makeup and remove contact lenses and dentures for surgery. *Do not put any moisturizer on your eyes or face.*
- Do not bring any jewelry or valuables. Wear a robe, housecoat or warmup suit that buttons or zips in the front, and wear flat shoes. *No tight-fitting clothes.*
- *Someone must drive you home and stay with you the first night.*
- Postoperative instructions regarding activity, medications and office visits will be given following your surgery.

THE SURGERY

If you have eyebrows that sit too low or droop too close to the eye, you'll want to consider a brow-lift. The surgery takes approximately one hour. Add an additional half hour for preparation and anesthesia. There are normally four people in the operating room with you: the surgeon, the anesthesiologist and two surgical nurses.

An incision is made either at the hairline or one or two finger-widths behind the hairline. If you like the option of wearing your hair away from your face, it's a better choice to request the incision behind the hairline, if it's surgically acceptable to your doctor and will produce the desired visual results. Always discuss the placement of incision lines with your doctor before surgery so you won't be surprised and unhappy with the choice of placement when you wake up and it's too late.

The incision usually runs a length of six to eight centimeters, depending on the amount and direction of lift the patient desires. In discussing the final results before surgery, be sure you understand exactly what the doctor has in mind. A brow- or coronal-lift that is pulled too high can leave you with a startled or surprised look—something you want to avoid at all costs. The skin is freed-up (separated from underlying tissues) from the incision down to the brow, then lifted to raise the center to the outer-tip portion of the brow up and back toward the high temple region.

Excess skin is trimmed and the incision is closed with stitches. The stitches are removed 12 to 14 days after surgery. It's important not to have the stitches removed too soon from a brow or a coronal lift. The pulling-up of the lift in these areas is so tight that unless the incision line is amply healed and secured, you could end up with a wide scar as a result of the incision's pulling apart from lack of stitch or staple support. So let your doctor take as much time as he wants before any stitch removal.

Another procedure, referred to as a Brow-Pexy, is also available as a separate choice to correct the drooping brow for male patients. The brow is lifted gently and actually secured to the brow bone. This procedure gives a mini-brow-lift result.

THE CORONAL-LIFT

If you have excessive forehead skin with deep lines across the forehead or loose skin between the brows above the nose, the full coronal-forehead-lift is the choice to make.

An incision called a coronal incision is made approximately four finger widths behind the hairline. The incision runs from one ear clear across the scalp to the other ear. The scalp and forehead skin are then freed up all the way down to the brows and lifted back up to the coronal incision line. The excess scalp and hair are trimmed away, and the incision is closed with a tight row of stainless steel surgical staples or with sutures.

Do not panic! I know the staples sound horrible, but they really don't hurt. Everything is so numb and tight-feeling up there for about 8 to 12 weeks following surgery that you will not feel more than a slight pulling sensation here and there. If your doctor closes your coronal incision with sutures, you'll still have a tight sensation in the area but it may be a little less severe than with the staples. It can be a bit unpleasant having the staples removed 12 to 14 days following surgery, but the removal is more annoying than painful. Don't be surprised if three or four of them are quite tender on the way out. It all goes very quickly, and once they're out you'll immediately begin to feel better and more relaxed. Following the removal, be sure to ask the nurse to double-check for any possible overlooked staples or sutures. It's easy to bypass a single staple or stitch here and there, and although it's not medically dangerous, it will save you an extra trip back into the office if they are all detected and removed at once.

Be sure to have a conversation with your doctor before surgery, insisting that the nurses who prep you the day of surgery either braid or separate your hair into sections to prevent horrendous tangling from blood coagulation into the hair. If that occurs, you may have to have chunks of hair cut out.

Muscles that produce wrinkles in the forehead and frown lines between the eyes can be severed at the time of coronal surgery to prevent them from returning or becoming more severe over time. However, a word of caution to actors: The cutting of muscles between the eyebrows can limit your facial movement and can therefore alter your range of expressions. You need to clearly discuss the pros and cons of this decision with your doctor before the actual surgery.

POSTSURGICAL INSTRUCTIONS

1. Rest quietly for one or two days. Then limit yourself to light activities. This means no housework heavier than rinsing a dish. Sleep with your head elevated for about 10 days.

2. Avoid straining, exercise or head-down positions, all of which may cause unnecessary swelling or bleeding.

3. Consider discomfort as an indication that you have been too active. REST! Take whatever prescribed medication your doctor has given you to help cut discomfort or to relax.

4. You may gently shampoo your hair with warm water right over the staples or sutures (baby shampoo or Neutrogena is preferred), beginning the day the dressing is removed, or sooner if no dressings were used. Ask your doctor exactly when you're allowed to shampoo. A shower is preferable to a bath in which the wound would be submerged.

THE RECOVERY PERIOD

You will be loosely bandaged for the 24 hours following surgery. A small amount of wound bleeding or ooze is natural for the first 48 hours.

Expect major numbness of the scalp and forehead for 8 to 12 weeks following the brow-lift or the coronal procedure. Swelling will occur immediately, leaving your forehead looking slightly inflated, and there will be a shiny quality to the skin. Don't worry—both symptoms usually disappear within the eight-week recovery period, leaving your forehead nice and taut with normal-looking skin.

Minimal bruising around and below the eyes will often occur with a brow- or coronal-lift; it usually disappears in three to eight weeks.

Following a coronal, you will experience a very tight feeling, like a bathing cap a couple of sizes too small. It normally passes within the 8- to 12-week recovery period, and you can usually ignore the tight sensation with the help of Tylenol. If you are a person prone to severe headaches or migraines, I strongly recommend you avoid coronal surgery. The constricted sensation over the head would probably be too uncomfortable for too many weeks. Choose another procedure if possible.

Expect the incision lines to raise up and turn bright pink before they flatten out and lose color. Often, just after the stitches or staples are removed, the incision line itself is so swollen it can create a slight separation in your hair. Because of this it is a good idea not to have your hair shorter than three or four inches before surgery. That way you have enough hair so that you can style some back over the separation.

As mentioned before, the coronal sutures must never be removed too early. There's so much tension on that particular incision that if the sutures are removed before 12 to 14 days post-op, you run a large risk of being left with a wide scar. Hair won't grow through a scar, and you'd have a permanent separation in your hair. This is the kind of problem you want to avoid.

Expect major numbness over the entire scalp and forehead for about 8 to 12 weeks. *Be very careful* when using electric appliances like hair dryers or curling irons during your numb period. Because you'll have no way of judging the heat, you could seriously burn your scalp without realizing it. Use all appliances on a low setting until your normal sensation returns.

Expect a loss of hair. You have had at least a one-inch strip cut out of your scalp and hair in order to pull everything up. Therefore, you'll have that much less hair on your head overall. Thick-haired people usually don't miss the loss, but it is something to be aware of if you have thin, fine hair. Know too that your hairline will be a little higher than it was before surgery. If you have an extremely high forehead, you may want to avoid coronal surgery.

PROBLEM SIGNS

Call your doctor at once if there is excessive bleeding from incision lines.

Occasionally a patient is left with permanent numbness around and near the incision line. It doesn't happen often, but it can happen.

MAKEUP TRICKS

About a week after the stitches or staples have been removed, you can camouflage any red incision lines in your hair by gently applying a soft eyebrow pencil in a color close to your hair color.

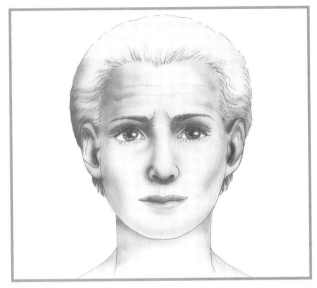

If your eyebrows sit too close to the eye, or you have drooping upper eyelids and deep furrows on your forehead, you'll want to consider a brow- or coronal-lift.

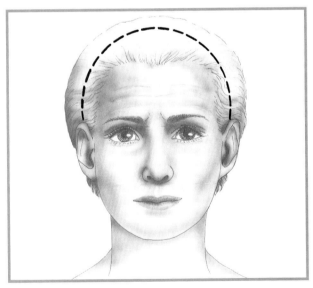

The coronal incision is usually four finger widths behind the hairline, with the incision running across the scalp. The scalp and forehead skin are then "freed up" all the way down to the brows and lifted back up to the incision line. The excess scalp is trimmed away, and the incision is closed with a row of surgical staples or width sutures.

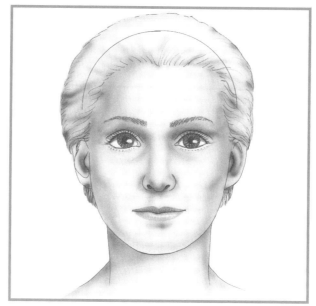

The finished results will leave you with a smooth forehead and brows that are repositioned into a slightly higher angle, framing upper lids that are now open.

CHAPTER TEN

Endoscopic Plastic Surgery

• • •

APPROXIMATE COST:

Eyebrow/Forehead-Lift: $3,500

Face-lift: $6,500

Breast Augmentation: $5,500

Abdominoplasty: $5,500

There may be additional charges for surgical facilities and anesthesia. Be sure to request this information.

Plastic surgery has adapted many of the endoscopic techniques that have been developed in gynecological, orthopedic, general and thoracic surgery. Theoretically, the endoscopic procedures result in less surgical trauma, smaller incisions and faster healing. Plastic surgeons are currently in the process of comparing many of the endoscopic techniques to the open surgical procedures, attempting to establish their effect on cost, operative risk and lasting results.

The endoscope is a telescope-like instrument that gives the plastic surgeon a window through which to see the anatomy and accomplish many of the cosmetic surgical procedures. The resulting scars are usually much smaller and often more satisfactory in appearance than the scars from traditional open surgical procedures. The most popular endoscopic procedures done through these relatively inconspicuous incisions are: the eyebrow / forehead-lift, face-lift, breast augmentation and abdominoplasty.

Endoscopic surgery involves the use of a fiber-optic light source and video camera introduced through one small incision. Instruments introduced through additional incisions allow the surgeon to remove tissue and to suture, staple and rearrange tissue. The majority of the procedure is observed on a television monitor, where the image has been transmitted from the endoscope.

ENDOSCOPIC EYEBROW / FOREHEAD-LIFT

The endoscopic eyebrow / forehead-lift was the first endoscopic plastic surgery technique developed. The procedure usually takes one to two hours; the surgical team includes your doctor and anesthesiologist, a surgical nurse and possibly a nurse technician. In chapter 4, I already described the traditional open surgical method, with its incision spanning from ear to ear. With the endoscopic approach, only three small incisions are made in the scalp. Through these incisions, the forehead skin is elevated and the eyebrows are freed-up from their attachment to the orbital bone. This procedure allows the eyebrows to be repositioned at a higher level on the forehead. The eyebrow elevation is maintained in position by using special sutures or miniscrews in the scalp incision. The screws or sutures are removed once the eyebrows have healed in their new position—usually two or more weeks after surgery. At the time of the eyebrow-lift, the frown muscles between the eyebrows can be weakened or removed (as they can be with a traditional coronal-lift). This additional correction seems to be one of the most popular reasons for having the endoscopic forehead surgery.

ENDOSCOPIC FACE-LIFT

An endoscopic face-lift usually takes three to four hours. The surgical team includes your doctor, the anesthesiologist, surgical nurses and perhaps a nurse technician.

Endoscopic face-lift procedures have been accomplished in two very different ways. The first is the subcutaneous, or more superficial, approach. This consists of elevating the skin through incisions at the hairline level and pulling the loose skin as a "pleat." The pleats are placed at the hairline level above or behind the ear, and slowly disappear over a period of several weeks.

The second endoscopic face-lift procedure lifts the deep structure of the face much in the same way that the eyebrows are lifted, by releasing or freeing up their attachment anchoring them to the facial bones. These structures are then secured at a higher, pulled-back position. Because the end result of lift and correction obtained in endoscopic face-lift surgery may be considerably less than that of the traditional face-lift procedure, patients with a lot of saggy or droopy skin, especially in the neck region, should definitely opt for a traditional face-lift.

ENDOSCOPIC BREAST SURGERY

Endoscopic breast surgery is an extension of current augmentation techniques, as well as an innovation in breast-lift procedures. Current breast augmentation via the armpit can often be accomplished more accurately with the endoscope. With endoscopy, breast implants may be inserted through an incision in the belly button (umbilicus). Small breasts can be lifted off the chest wall and repositioned at a higher level, all done through the armpit or with an incision around the perimeter of the nipple area. A modest degree of breast reduction can be accomplished in a similar manner through small incisions around the nipple area or through the armpit.

ENDOSCOPIC ABDOMINOPLASTY

Endoscopic abdominoplasty usually takes three to four hours. Your doctor, an anesthesiologist, surgical nurses and a nurse technician may be in the operating room with you during the procedure. Endoscopic abdominoplasty is now available for young women with a mild amount of abdominal laxity. Through small incisions in the pubic area, the endoscopic correction is performed in conjunction with liposuction of the abdomen and flanks. If you have severe amounts of loose abdominal skin, you will want to choose the traditional open surgical procedure for abdominoplasty, as the endoscopic technique would probably not give a sufficient result.

Whether you are having a cosmetic procedure performed by endoscopic or open technique, the same preoperative and postoperative precautions and considerations apply. The use of anti-swelling techniques and cosmetics for bruises is likely to apply to some degree in all cases. If you qualify, endoscopic surgical techniques may offer a distinct advantage in expediting healing and minimizing scarring. But if you're trying to correct saggy skin around the neck area, choose a traditional face-lift.

CHAPTER ELEVEN

Breast Augmentation

• • •

APPROXIMATE COST: $2,600–$5,588

There may be additional charges for surgical facilities and anesthesia. Be sure to request this information.

APPROXIMATE TIME UNTIL COMPLETELY HEALED:

One to three months. The scars will take at least a year to fade out to their minimal color.

BEFORE YOU SET A DATE

Prior to surgery be sure you meet with your doctor at least three times to be absolutely certain that you are both clear and in agreement as to your choice of incision lines and the desired shape and size of the breasts you envision. The best way to communicate the type of breast you want is to bring in pictures from *Playboy* or other men's magazines that exemplify your desired final results.

Saline inflatable implants are presently the only legally available breast implants. There are a couple of problems with these implants, though, that you should be aware of. First, because there is a valve involved, the saline can leak out. This is not medically dangerous. But as the saline leaks the breast will become smaller, eventually requiring another surgical procedure to replace the fluid and correct the diminished size. You should know that with saline inflatable implants, the possibility of more surgeries for adjustments does exist. If silicone implants stay off the market, the saline implant manufacturers will most likely produce an implant without a valve, eliminating this leakage problem.

The other problem that you'd best be aware of is that you can actually hear the saline sloshing around a bit with pronounced movement, particularly if the implant is placed above the pectoral muscle.

The first decision you and your doctor will make concerns placement of the incision line through which the implant will be inserted. You have three choices: under the armpit, in the crease under the breast where it meets the body or around the lower half of the nipple base (the areola).

Implanting through the armpit has become quite popular, but you will be left with a slight visible scar, and apparently there's some real discomfort upon awakening from anesthesia. The muscles under the arm tend to spasm, but a little pain medication will get you through very nicely until the spasms pass.

Implanting through the under-breast crease is also fine, but it will leave a visible scar when you're lying down.

Entrance through the lower part of the nipple-base seems to be the best bet for the least noticeable scar. Women who have never had children often have very small nipples, which can limit the doctor's access. However, the inflatable implant seems to work nicely in these cases.

The second decision you must make, with the advice of your surgeon, is whether the implant should be placed under or above the pectoral (breast) muscle. Normally surgeons prefer to have as much tissue as possible covering the implant, so they tend to want to place it under the muscle. The downside to this choice is that it can be quite uncomfortable for three or four days following surgery. But so what? If it's the better choice for your overall end result, it is reasonable to decide to control the discomfort with pain medication for a few days.

If you're a middle-aged woman who has nursed children and has sagging breasts, it is advisable to place the saline implant above the muscle. The implant would raise the hanging breast up into a more attractive position. If for some reason this choice is not possible, the fallen breast type of patient could have the implant placed below the breast muscle and also have breast-reduction surgery. But why go through two separate procedures if it's not necessary?

If you're a very thin woman, it is not advisable to place the implant above the muscle. In thin women the implants seem too obvious and detectable unless they are placed under the muscle, with the extra tissue coverage to soften the final look of the breast.

Athletes with highly developed pectoral muscles, such as swimmers, gymnasts or weightlifters, may not be good candidates for implants. If placed below an extremely developed muscle, the implant just doesn't look natural, and when positioned above a developed muscle it looks fake and severe.

It's very important to carefully discuss implant placement with your doctor before surgery to ensure that you'll make the appropriate choice for your lifestyle.

PRESURGICAL INSTRUCTIONS

- You will be given blood and lab tests approximately two weeks prior to your surgery. X-rays and a mammogram will be taken prior to surgery. Take no aspirin or aspirin-containing products; they can cause bleeding and bruising. See list of medications to avoid for two weeks prior to your surgery and one week after. You may take Tylenol.

- If you take medication daily, notify your doctor. Also inform him if you develop an illness, a cold or any skin infections within a week of your surgery.

- If you're a smoker you should clearly understand that nicotine can impair and delay healing. Most offices will suggest quitting a week to 10 days before surgery, a week post-op. If it were me, I'd stop smoking a minimum of three weeks prior to surgery, and not touch a cigarette for a full month post-op. Who needs to be left with scars worse than normal and other complications as a result of smoking through the pre- and postsurgical period?

THE DAY BEFORE SURGERY

Do not eat or drink anything after midnight.

THE DAY OF SURGERY

- You may rinse and brush your teeth, but *do not eat or drink anything.* Some offices may ask you take pills with a small amount of water the day of surgery. Do not bring any jewelry or valuables. Wear a robe, housecoat or warmup suit that buttons or zips in the front, and wear flat shoes. *No tight-fitting clothes.*

- *Someone must drive you home the day of your surgery and stay with you the first night.*

- Postoperative instructions regarding activity, medications and office visits will be given following your surgery.

THE SURGERY

A breast augmentation usually takes an hour and a half to two hours. Add an additional half hour for preparation and anesthesia. There are normally four people in the operating room with you: the surgeon, the anesthesiologist and two surgical nurses. You will be given an intravenous anesthetic. Antibiotics will also be administered through the I.V. to protect against infection.

Entrance to the breast area is made through one of the choices previously discussed: under the arm, the crease under the breast or the bottom half of the nipple base. Working through the incision, the doctor lifts the breast tissue up and pushes the skin down to create a pocket either under the breast muscle or above it, depending on your choice of implant placement.

The incision lines are closed with sutures.

POSTSURGICAL INSTRUCTIONS

1. Rest at home for one or two days following surgery. Then engage in only very light activity for at least 10 days.

2. Continue antibiotics as directed following your surgery. If diarrhea develops, discontinue the antibiotic and contact the doctor's office.

3. If you have been given ibuprofen (Motrin), eat bland foods and discontinue the ibuprofen if an abdominal burning pain or nausea develops.

4. Take Vitamin E 4000 I.U. per day for six weeks followed by 2000 I.U. per day for one year.

5. Do not resume aspirin products for at least 10 days after surgery.

6. Wear a supportive bra 24 hours a day for six weeks. (Remove bra to shower).*

7. Approximately seven days after your breast surgery, a return to the office for suture removal will be scheduled. Some doctors use absorbable sutures that will dissolve on their own.

8. Strenuous activity such as sports, aerobics and any type of manual labor should be curtailed for one month. Activity of the upper extremities should be restricted to the limits of comfort for six weeks. Avoid lifting anything more than five pounds for the first two weeks following surgery. No driving, no sudden movements, no heavy housework, no reaching for top shelves for at least 10 days. If you blow your hair dry, keep the dryer at a low angle for a couple of weeks. Thereafter, gradually resume normal activity.

* *These instructions may vary with your individual case. Clarify these items with your doctor.*

THE RECOVERY PERIOD

You will probably experience some pain the first three to four days following surgery and remain sore for about two weeks. Pain medication will help you through the first four days, and Tylenol should ease the remaining soreness. Swelling and bruising usually clears up within two or three weeks. The incision lines will raise up and turn bright pink for several weeks.

PROBLEM SIGNS

If there is any bleeding via the incision lines or any indication of infection, call your doctor at once. Look for ballooning, pinkness, warmness, tightness and swelling as problem signs. Any pain could indicate blood clots that would require surgical removal.

Be aware that no woman's breasts are perfectly matched; there are always differences in size and shape. Most breast augmentation procedures may enhance these differences, even if your surgeon uses different-sized implants. While healing from surgery, asymmetry of the breasts may occur due to one side healing differently than the other. If so, an additional surgery would be required to correct the problem.

If your scars begin to really thicken and turn red, you may be developing a keloid, which is a severe thickening of scar tissue. Call your doctor *immediately*. He will give you a cortisone cream or tape to apply to the scar, or he'll use an injection that will most probably correct the problem. If you wait too long, the scar won't be correctable, so report the problem as soon as you see it.

Some hardness may develop in the months following surgery. Your doctor may instruct you on a program of breast massage to induce softening. With breast implants, you run the risk of excessive scar tissue forming around the implant. This is called "capsular contracture," and it causes the breast to become unnaturally hard. A second surgery is required to correct this problem.

Any breast implants impair the detection of possible breast cancer via mammograms, X-rays and so forth. The technician must carefully displace the implant in order to take an X-ray.

MAKEUP TRICKS

If your scars are completely healed and dry they may be safely camouflaged approximately one week following suture removal with a foundation that matches your skin tone. Dermablend; Physicians Formula Velvet Film; Max Factor Pan Stick; Clinique Continuous Coverage or Prescriptives Camouflage Creme, Cover Mark or Natural Cover all are good choices for scar coverage.

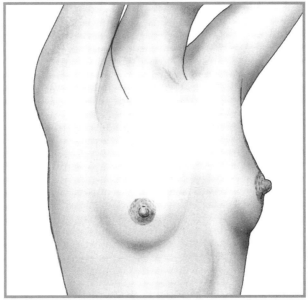

If you feel your breasts are too small in size, you may opt for breast augmentation.

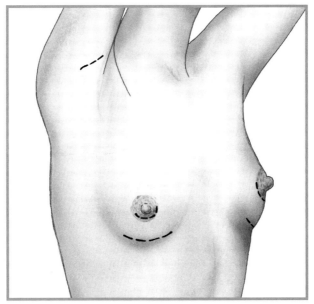

Incisions can be made in one of three places: under the arm, in the crease under the breast, or in the bottom half of the nipple base.

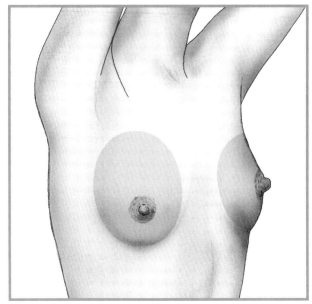

Pockets are created in the shaded area to receive the implants.

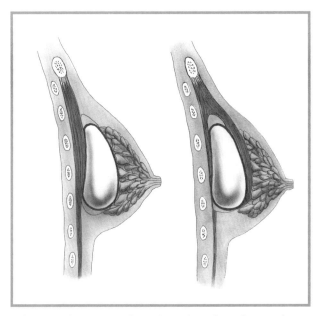

The implant can be placed either beneath or above the pectoral muscle.

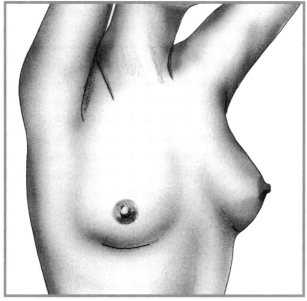

The final results: fuller breasts that should appear natural in size, shape and color.

CHAPTER TWELVE

Breast Reduction

• • •

APPROXIMATE COST: $4,600–$7,975

There may be additional charges for surgical facilities and anesthesia. Be sure to request this information.

APPROXIMATE TIME UNTIL COMPLETELY HEALED:

One to three months. The scars will take at least a year to fade out to their minimal color.

PRESURGICAL INSTRUCTIONS

- You will be given blood and lab tests prior to surgery. Your doctor will send you for X-rays and mammograms. Do not take any aspirin or aspirin-containing products; they can cause bleeding and bruising. See list of medications to avoid for two weeks prior to your surgery and one week after. You may take Tylenol.

- If you take medication daily, notify your doctor. Also inform him if you develop an illness, a cold or any skin infections within a week of your surgery.

- Take an iron supplement at least one month prior to surgery, as well as one month afterward.

- If you're a smoker you should clearly understand that nicotine can impair and delay healing. Most offices will suggest quitting a week to 10 days before surgery and a week after. If it were me, I'd stop smoking a minimum of three weeks prior to surgery and not touch a cigarette for a full month post-op. Who needs to be left with scars worse than normal and other complications as a result of smoking through the pre- and postsurgical period?

THE DAY BEFORE SURGERY

Do not eat or drink anything after midnight.

THE DAY OF SURGERY

- You may rinse and brush your teeth, but *do not eat or drink anything*. Some offices may ask you to take pills with a small amount of water the day of the surgery. Do not bring any jewelry or valuables. Wear a robe, housecoat or warmup suit that buttons or zips in the front, and wear flat shoes. *No tight-fitting clothes.*

- *Someone must drive you home and stay with you the first night.*

- Postoperative instructions regarding activity, medications and office visits will be given following your surgery.

THE SURGERY

The surgery takes about three hours. Add an additional half hour for preparation and anesthesia. There are usually four people in the operating room with you: the surgeon, the anesthesiologist and two surgical nurses.

Breast reduction is exactly what it implies: it reduces the size and shape of large, hanging breasts, and reduces the nipple size if necessary. It relieves the weight-induced pain in the breasts, neck, shoulders and back, and enhances your appearance by giving your body more balanced proportions.

Before the operation you must carefully explain to your doctor exactly how you would like to look as a result of your reduction surgery. Bring in pictures from *Playboy* and other men's magazines to demonstrate your choices.

Horizontal and vertical incisions that follow the breast contour are made, with a circular incision at the top of the vertical section to receive the nipple once the breast is lifted up. Working through the incisions, the surgeon removes excess fat, tissue and skin, along with the skin within the vertical section. If the nipple needs reducing, the skin around the areola (nipple base) is also removed. The nipple and breast are lifted up and repositioned to the new nipple site, and the skin on both sides of the breast is brought down and around the areola, then sutured together to reshape the breast. You will have sutures around the entire areola, straight down the bottom half of the breast, and clear across the under-breast crease. The sutures will often be covered with steri-strips for additional support. The sutures and steri-strips will be removed in two weeks.

An alternative surgical process is to fully detach the nipple and nipple base from the breast and then surgically relocate it. However, a transplanted nipple becomes totally void of feeling and sensation, so most doctors prefer to avoid this procedure if possible.

POSTSURGICAL INSTRUCTIONS

1. Rest quietly for one or two days, then engage in only very light activity for at least 10 days.

2. Continue antibiotics as directed following your surgery. If diarrhea develops, discontinue the antibiotics and contact the office.

3. If you have been given ibuprofen (Motrin), eat bland foods and discontinue the ibuprofen if an abdominal burning pain or nausea develops.

4. Take Vitamin E 4000 I.U. per day for six weeks followed by 2000 I.U. per day for one year.

5. Do not resume aspirin products for at least 10 days after surgery.

6. Wear a supportive bra 24 hours a day for six weeks. (Remove bra to shower.)*

7. You may shower over the stitches and steri-strips, gently patting dry.

8. Approximately seven days after your breast surgery, a return to the office for suture removal will be scheduled.*

9. Strenuous activity (sports, aerobics, manual labor) should be curtailed for one month. Activity of the upper extremities should be restricted to the limits of comfort for six weeks. Avoid lifting anything more than five pounds for the first two weeks following surgery. No driving, no sudden movements, no heavy housework, no reaching for top shelves for at least 10 days. If you blow your hair dry, keep the dryer at a low angle for a couple of weeks. Thereafter, gradually resume normal activity.

* *These instructions may vary with your individual case. Clarify these items with your doctor.*

THE RECOVERY PERIOD

You'll experience some pain during the first three or four days; it can be managed with prescribed medication. You'll remain sore for about three to four weeks, and Tylenol should get you through that period. You'll be wearing a surgical bra for support for six weeks post-op.

Any swelling and bruising should pass within two or three weeks. The scars will raise up and turn bright pink before flattening out. Expect the scars to be extremely obvious for a year post-op. They will eventually begin to fade a bit, but they will always remain apparent. It's a trade off: beautifully sized and shaped breasts, but with permanent scars. However, all of these scars will be completely undetectable under a bra, bathing suit or strapless evening dress.

Wait at least three weeks for the swelling to subside before you run out and purchase a new bra wardrobe.

PROBLEM SIGNS

If there is any bleeding from incision lines or indications of infection, call your doctor immediately. Severe pain could indicate blood clots that will need to be surgically removed. Any ballooning, pinkness, warmness, tingling or excessive swelling should be considered a possible problem.

If any incision line really thickens up and turns red, you may be developing a keloid. See your doctor *immediately* for treatment. Don't wait! The scar needs instant attention.

If you notice any remarkable asymmetry developing, call your doctor and have him examine you A.S.A.P.

MAKEUP TRICKS

If your scars are completely healed and dry, they may be safely camouflaged approximately one week following suture removal with a foundation that matches your skin tone. Dermablend, Physicians Formula Velvet Film, Max Factor Pan Stick, Clinique's Continuous Coverage, Cover Mark, Prescriptives Camouflage Creme or Natural Cover all are good choices for scar coverage.

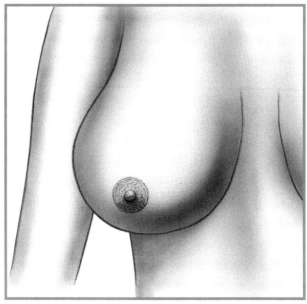

If you feel the size and shape of your breast is too large or sagging, breast reduction is a procedure to consider.

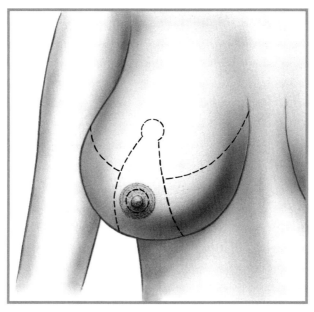

Horizontal and vertical incisions are made with a top circular incision to receive the nipple once the breast is lifted up.

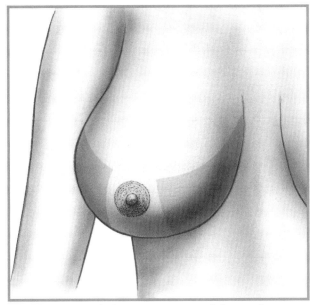

Fat, tissue and skin are removed from the shaded areas.

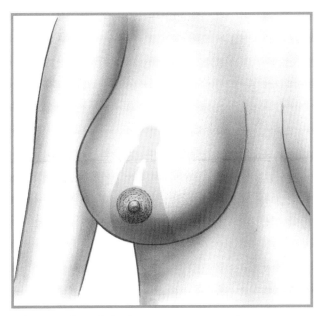

The nipple is lifted up into its new location.

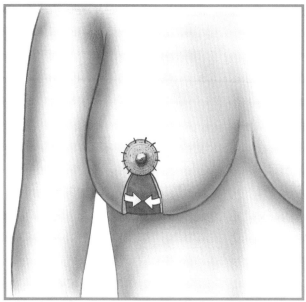

The skin that was positioned above the original nipple site is brought down and together to the breast.

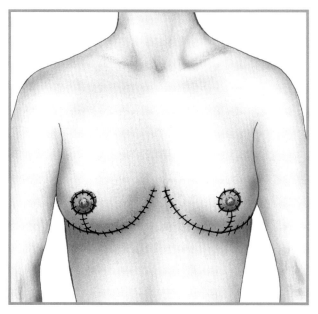

Sutures are placed around the entire areola, down the bottom half of the breast, and across the under-breast crease.

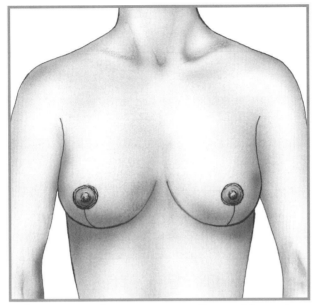

*After surgery, breasts are smaller and beauti-
fully shaped.*

CHAPTER THIRTEEN

Breast Implant Removal

• • •

APPROXIMATE COST:

Implant removal only: $1,000

Implant removal and saline implant exchange: $2,000

Implant removal with removal
of capsular contracture: $2,000–$3,000

Implant removal with saline implant exchange
and removal of capsular contracture: $3,000–$4,000

Obviously, there exists a tremendous amount of controversy about silicone gel implants. If you are experiencing capsular contracture (a hardening of the breast due to a fibrous capsule the body has formed around the implant, often causing pain), you will want to remove the implants. Other possible reasons for implant removal include a ruptured implant (you might notice a change in the shape and feel of the breast with implant rupture); breast cancer detection may be too difficult; concern over autoimmune symptoms you believe to be silicone related; infection; granulomas (nonmalignant lumps that form around drops of silicone); breast pain or just a desire to have the implants removed.

A great deal has been written about the possible link between silicone gel and autoimmune disease. The symptoms include joint swelling and pain, severe fatigue, headaches and skin rashes, to name a few. If you are suffering from these symptoms, the first thing to do is see a qualified rheumatologist for a complete workup. The findings of this workup will assist in determining whether or not you should have the implants removed.

The majority of physicians do not believe that silicone gel causes autoimmune disease. No one, however, really knows the specifics yet. This also applies to the subject of cancer caused by silicone. Both possibilities are hypothetical and will require continued medical monitoring.

THE SURGERY

Implant removal is done under a general anesthetic. An incision is made either under the breast crease or around the bottom half of the areola (nipple base). The surgeon enters the breast through one of these sites and carefully slips the implant out of the body. The scar tissue around the implant is removed wherever possible to reduce any "spillover" silicone in the breast region. The breast pocket is then irrigated and sutured closed. Occasionally a drain tube is required for a few days.

If the implant has ruptured, the surgery becomes quite extensive in attempts to remove as much of the gel as possible. During silicone implant removal, many patients opt to have saline inflatable implants substituted into the site at the time of surgery. Don't forget that saline inflatable implants will deflate with time, requiring more surgery to reinflate them. Also, thin patients can hear the saline implants slosh.

Some people opt for no replacement at all following implant removal. For women on the thin side, be prepared to be really unhappy with the results. There will be a severe loss of volume, probable distortion and wrinkling. Your breasts will look far worse than before your implant surgery. In some cases, further reconstruction is impossible because of scar contractures.

Patients with significant amounts of fat and tissue beneath the breast will probably find themselves feeling quite comfortable without implant replacement.

Mastectomy reconstruction patients have great success with rebuilding from the abdominal tissues into the breast area. This requires more complicated surgery and permanent scars on the abdomen, but the results are excellent (see chapter 14).

Which decision to take following implant removal is an extremely difficult and personal judgment call. Discuss your options at length with your doctor before undergoing surgery.

CHAPTER FOURTEEN

Post-Mastectomy Reconstruction

• • •

APPROXIMATE COST:

Reconstruction: $6,738

Nipple reduction: $3,488

There may be additional charges for surgical facilities and anesthesia. Be sure to request this information.

APPROXIMATE TIME UNTIL COMPLETELY FINISHED
WITH THE PROCESS AND HEALED:

One to two years.

BEFORE YOU SET A DATE

It is critical that you understand that this is not an elective procedure designed to make you look more attractive and alluring. Breast reconstruction following a mastectomy should be approached as a possibly fatal medical problem. In other words, never allow your aesthetic desires for your reconstructed breast to outweigh the medical aspects of the disease. The treatment for breast cancer is not geared to the aesthetics of reconstructive surgery, and therapies to eliminate the cancer must take precedence over the appearance of your breast.

You should first find a properly qualified cancer surgeon and discuss precisely what is the best mode of medical treatment for your individual case. Then you can approach a plastic surgeon and decide how to aesthetically correct the damage following the proper medical treatment.

PRESURGICAL INSTRUCTIONS

- You will be given blood and lab tests prior to surgery. Your doctor will send you for X-rays and mammograms. Do not take aspirin or aspirin-containing products; they can cause bleeding and bruising. See list of medications to avoid for two weeks prior to your surgery and one week after. You may take Tylenol.

- If you take medication daily, notify your doctor. Also tell him if you develop an illness, cold or any skin infections within a week of your surgery.

- Take an iron supplement at least one month prior to surgery, as well as one month afterward.

- If you're a smoker you should clearly understand that nicotine can impair and delay healing. Most offices will suggest quitting a week to 10 days before surgery, and a week post-op. If it were me, I'd stop smoking a minimum of three weeks prior to surgery and not touch a cigarette for a full month post-op. Who needs to be left with scars worse than normal and other complications as a result of smoking through the pre- and postsurgical period?

THE DAY BEFORE SURGERY

Do not eat or drink anything after midnight.

THE DAY OF SURGERY

- You may rinse and brush your teeth, but *do not eat or drink anything.* Some offices may ask you to take pills with a small amount of water the day of surgery.

- Do not wear any jewelry or bring valuables. Wear a robe, housecoat or warmup suit that buttons or zips in the front, and wear flat shoes. *No tight-fitting clothing.*

- *Someone must drive you home and stay with you the first night.*

- Postoperative instructions regarding activity, medications and office visits will be given following your surgery.

THE SURGERY

There are usually four people in the operating room with you: the surgeon, the anesthesiologist and two surgical nurses. Your cancer specialist may also choose to be present, and additional nurses may be utilized. You will be given a general anesthetic intravenously, as well as an I.V. antibiotic. The mastectomy with breast reconstruction takes about three to four hours.

A modified radical mastectomy involves the removal of the breast, nipple and areola, and the lymph glands in the axilla (armpit). Breast reconstruction procedures can usually follow in the same surgery. This original procedure always takes place in the hospital.

An incision is made where the lower breast would exist, and the skin and underlying muscle are raised to create a pocket to receive a saline inflatable implant. The implant is not fully inflated, because that would create too much tension on the wound. A reservoir is left under the skin, and after the wounds are fully healed the surgeon can inflate the implant and stretch out the tissues by injecting a needle into the implant through the skin.

At a later date, usually three to six months after your original surgery, this temporary implant is removed and an appropriate shaping of the pocket and placement of a regular full implant is made. Sutures are removed from the incision line at the breast base seven days post-op. At this time the patient with an intact healthy breast should decide what, if any, surgery to undergo so that the two breasts will match. If the remaining breast is large and drooping or small and flat, you might want to consider reshaping it as well. Your ultimate goal is symmetry.

Sometimes, due to the nature or the location of the tumor, large amounts of skin must be removed or the skin on the chest is too tight to receive an implant. The surgeon is then faced with the problem of replacing the skin as well as recreating a breast mound.

The most common approach is to use the tissue in the lower abdomen, which is basically the same skin and fat that is discarded in a tummy tuck. This technique is called the TRAM procedure, and it also requires a three-to-six month healing period from the original surgery before it can be performed.

Incisions are made in the apron of the lower abdomen to form a flap consisting of part of the rectus abdominous muscle and its overlying skin and fat. The flap is channeled up through the abdomen to the chest wall, creating shape to the breast without the use of an implant. Sutures are used to secure the new tissue, and the incision on the abdomen is sutured closed. Sometimes dissolvable stitches which require no removal will be used. If skin stitches are used, they must remain in at least 7 to 10 days, but no longer than 14 days post-op. Abdominal stitches come out 14 days following surgery.

Another transplant procedure involves taking the tissue from the back. However, there's usually not enough fat in the back area to allow breast reconstruction without the additional use of an implant. The back tissue is transplanted to the breast area by channeling the muscle, skin and fat under the skin and around the side of the body to the mastectomy site. It is sutured to the existing breast skin to create a pocket to receive a saline implant. The incision on the back is sutured closed. The sutures on the breast are removed seven days post-op. The stitches on the back will come out 7 to 10 days after surgery.

Another reconstructive procedure involves placing a balloon-like device called a tissue expander under the chest muscle and gradually filling it with saline over a period of several weeks. The skin stretches to form a breast mound. The expander can usually be implanted three to six months following the original surgery.

A new technique is free-flap transfer. This procedure utilizes tissue from the abdomen, buttocks or back. The donor tissue, including the artery and vein, is completely removed. It's then reconnected to the breast area, and the artery and vein are joined to the vascular network (generally in the armpit).

The decision to use this technique or the others mentioned is based upon your anatomy, your operative site and your surgeon's experience.

Following completion of mound reconstruction, nipple and areola reconstruction can begin. Skin grafts, most commonly from the inner thigh and from the lips of the vagina, are used to construct a new nipple and areola. Tattoo can be used later to permanently color the nipple.

All of the above procedures involve a series of surgeries that take a total of one to two years. It's a slow process that requires complete healing between procedures.

So you're going to have to be enormously patient, but think of it this way: Although you will have some permanent scars that will be covered up in a bra or a bathing suit, you will have a very nice shape and contour as a result of reconstruction.

POSTSURGICAL INSTRUCTIONS

1. Rest quietly for one or two days, then engage in only very light activity for at least 10 days.

2. Continue antibiotics as directed following your surgery. If diarrhea develops, discontinue the antibiotic and contact the doctor's office.

3. If you have been given ibuprofen (Motrin), eat bland foods. Discontinue the ibuprofen if an abdominal burning pain or nausea develops.

4. Take Vitamin E 4000 I.U. per day for six weeks followed by 2000 I.U. per day for one year.

5. Do not resume aspirin products for at least 10 days after surgery.

6. Wear a supportive bra 24 hours a day for six weeks. (Remove bra to shower.)*

7. You may shower over the stitches and steri-strips, gently patting dry.

8. Approximately seven days after your breast surgery, a return to the office for suture removal will be scheduled.*

9. Strenuous activity (sports, aerobics, manual labor) should be curtailed for one month. Activity of the upper extremities should be restricted to the limits of comfort for six weeks. Avoid lifting anything more than five pounds for the first two weeks following surgery. No driving, no sudden movements, no heavy housework, no reaching for top shelves for at least 10 days. If you

blow your hair dry, keep the dryer at a low angle for a couple of weeks. Thereafter, gradually resume normal activity.

*   *These instructions may vary with your individual case. Clarify these items with your doctor.*

THE RECOVERY PERIOD

You've just gone through some extremely serious surgery and an emotionally rough time as well. Expect to experience a combination of major relief and depression. You'll be exhausted for the first several days. For the first three to four days any pain can be controlled with medication. Expect to remain very tender for several weeks; take Tylenol to help you through this phase. You'll be wearing a surgical bra for support for several weeks post-op.

Any swelling and bruising should pass in three to five weeks. The scars will raise up and turn bright pink before they flatten out. Expect the scars to remain obvious even after they flatten out and lose color. The reconstructed breast will feel firmer than a normal breast, and it will not exactly match your healthy breast in shape. Expect some sensation to return to the breast area.

Post-mastectomy reconstruction has no effect on the possible recurrence of breast cancer.

PROBLEM SIGNS

If you have any bleeding from incisions or signs of infection, call your doctor immediately. Severe pain could indicate blood clots that would require surgical removal. Any ballooning, tingling, warmness or excessive swelling should be reported to your doctor.

An additional surgery may be necessary to revise scars or soften breasts that have become too firm as a result of excess scar tissue.

MAKEUP TRICKS

If your scars are completely healed and dry, they may be safely camouflaged approximately one week following suture removal with a foundation that matches your skin tone. Dermablend, Physicians Formula Velvet film, Max Factor Pan Stick, Clinique Continuous Coverage, Prescriptives Camouflage Creme, Cover Mark or Natural Cover all are good choices for scar coverage.

POST-MASTECTOMY RECONSTRUCTION

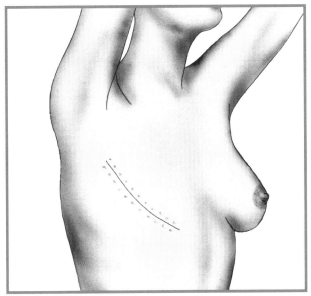

Once you have completely recovered from your mastectomy, you can proceed with breast reconstruction.

POST-MASTECTOMY RECONSTRUCTION WITH SALINE IMPLANT

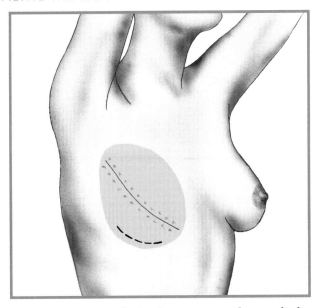

An incision is made in the crease underneath the breast, and the shaded area including the pectoral muscles are freed-up to form a pocket that will hold the implant.

POST-MASTECTOMY RECONSTRUCTION
WITH SALINE IMPLANT

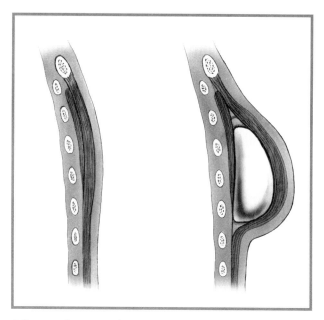

The implant is placed under the muscle.

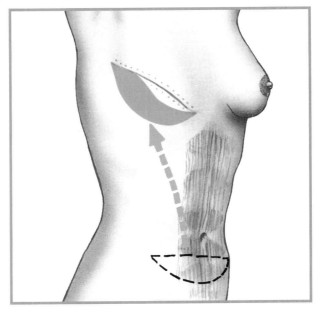

A skin flap consisting of muscle, skin and fat is taken from the abdominal apron.

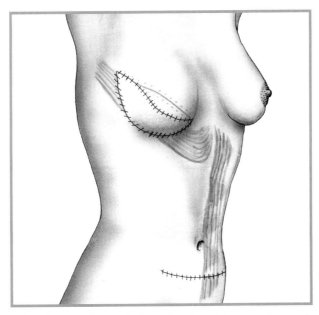

The flap is channeled under the skin, up through the abdominal wall to the mastectomy site.

POST-MASTECTOMY RECONSTRUCTION
WITH ABDOMINAL TRAM

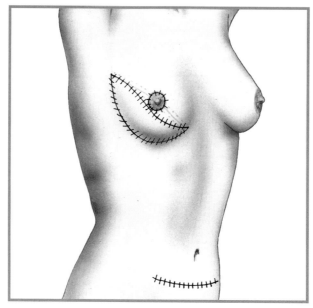

Following abdominal TRAM surgery and nipple reconstruction, the patient will be left with the indicated scars.

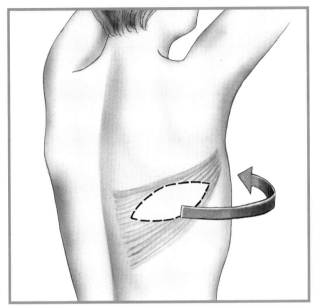

The back tissue and muscle are channeled under the skin to the mastectomy site.

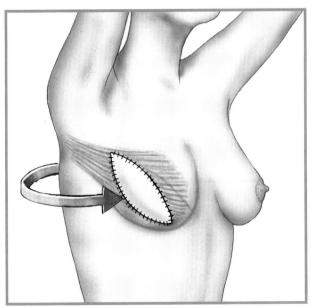

The tissue and muscle are sutured to the existing breast skin to create a pocket to receive a saline implant. The implant is placed in the newly formed pocket.

POST-MASTECTOMY RECONSTRUCTION
WITH BACK TISSUE TRANSPLANT

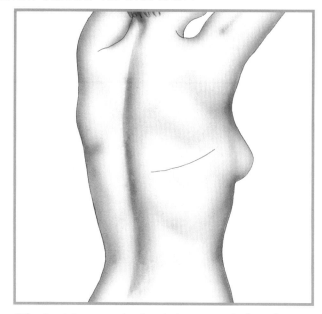

The incision on the back is sutured closed.

CHAPTER FIFTEEN

Liposuction

• • •

APPROXIMATE COST: $800–$4,600 *depending on targeted area.*

Additional charges may be required for surgical facilities and anesthesia. Be sure to request this information.

APPROXIMATE TIME UNTIL COMPLETELY HEALED:

Four to 12 weeks.

BEFORE YOU SET A DATE

Get very realistic about the results you can expect. Liposuction is good for moderately reducing fat in specific areas such as the hips, buttocks, thighs, abdomen and "love handles" above the waist. Fat removal from the arms, knee areas, above the breast and under the chin and neck is also quite successfully accomplished through this procedure. Fat suctioning in the calves must be done with great caution because most of the lower leg is bone and muscle and has only minimal amounts of actual fat.

Suctioning fat that is very close to the skin can leave you with wrinkling and cellulite. Easiest to remove are the deep fat pads that lie under a cushion of normal fat, as do the "saddle-bag" areas on the outer thighs or the stomach.

Cellulite cannot be removed with liposuction. Cellulite is caused by the fibrous connections between the skin and the fascia of the muscle; the attachments cause a dimpling of the skin. If your fat has "quilted" within these fibrous connections and you try to remove it with liposuction, the cellulite dimpling can actually appear worse.

Your surgeon's challenge is to remove as much fat as possible while leaving some fat between the skin as a cushion. If no cushion is left, you could end up with wrinkling, deformities and/or cellulite.

Liposuction can greatly improve the contour of your body, but it is *not* a cure for overweight bodies. There will be many remaining fat cells in the area that was liposuctioned. Your doctor cannot remove all the fat cells from an area without creating other problems. So understand that if you gain weight after liposuction, the remaining fat cells will expand and you'll look heavy again. Get it straight in your mind: Liposuction will not be transforming you into a wisp or a gazelle. Instead, your natural silhouette will look better.

PRESURGICAL INSTRUCTIONS

- You will be given blood and lab tests approximately two weeks prior to surgery. Take no aspirin or aspirin-containing products for two weeks prior to your surgery and 10 days after (see list of medications to avoid). You may take Tylenol.

- If you take medication daily, notify your doctor. Also tell him if you develop an illness or cold within a week of your surgery.

- If you're a smoker you should clearly understand that nicotine can impair and delay healing. Most offices will suggest quitting a week to 10 days before surgery, a week post-op. If it were me, I'd stop smoking a minimum of three weeks prior to surgery and not touch a cigarette for a full month post-op. Who needs to be left with scars worse than normal and other complications as a result of smoking through the pre- and postsurgical period?

THE DAY BEFORE SURGERY

Do not eat or drink anything after midnight. The night before or the morning of surgery, you can shower and shampoo your hair.

THE DAY OF SURGERY

- You may rinse and brush your teeth but do *not eat or drink anything.*

- Wear no makeup and remove contact lenses and dentures for surgery. *No moisturizer or body lotions.*

- Do not bring any jewelry or valuables. Wear a robe, housecoat or warmup suit that buttons or zips in the front, and wear flat shoes. No tight-fitting clothes.

- *Someone must drive you home and stay with you the first night.*

- Postoperative instructions regarding activity, medications and office visits will be given following your surgery.

THE SURGERY

The surgical time will vary depending on which areas you are having liposuctioned. The thigh and leg usually run about an hour and a half; the abdomen and flanks take approximately two hours. For whichever procedure you're having, add an additional half hour for preparation and anesthesia.

You will be given a general anesthetic. The surgery may also be performed under a local anesthetic to numb the specific area. If you're having a large area liposuctioned, and if general anesthesia is medically safe for you, you'll probably want to opt for the general for comfort's sake. Antibiotics will be given to you through an I.V. during surgery.

Small incisions (approximately half an inch long) are made in the area where liposuction will occur. For instance, the incision will be placed in the fold under the buttocks for access to upper thighs and buttocks. Question your doctor very carefully to be sure you know where each incision will be placed. You don't want surprise scars on your body.

A tubular instrument hooked up to a suction unit is inserted through the incisions, a high-vacuum pressure is created and the fat is suctioned out. The suctioning can also be done effectively with a syringe; your surgeon will decide which option is appropriate. The doctor will manipulate the tube in the tissue between the skin and the muscle fascia, removing the fat from the area.

At one time the recommended amount of fat to be removed at one sitting without getting blood transfusions was 1,500 cc (the equivalent of one pound of fat).

Today there is a new technique called tumescent liposuction. This technique infuses a physiologic solution into the area to be suctioned. The solution contains a local anesthetic to reduce pain, adhesions and bleeding. Using tumescent liposuction, the amount of fat that can safely be suctioned is increased to two or three pounds.

The incisions are sutured closed for seven days. You will be given a surgical girdle to help relieve swelling and discomfort. You must wear this girdle 24 hours a day for the first week post-op, and then, depending upon your swelling and bruising, your doctor will advise you how long to continue wearing this support.

POSTSURGICAL INSTRUCTIONS

1. Bed rest with legs elevated the day of surgery. From then on, physical activity should be limited to movements that are comfortable.

2. Wear the supportive garment that was selected prior to the surgery 24 hours a day for seven days or longer as instructed. As a general rule, the supportive garment should be worn until the bruising and discomfort have subsided, usually two or three weeks post-op.

3. Polysporin Ointment should be applied to the sutures daily until suture removal (approximately seven days). Use a cotton-tipped applicator to apply the ointment.

4. Continue the antibiotics as instructed. If you develop diarrhea, discontinue antibiotics and notify your doctor.

5. Anesthetics and pain medication tend to produce constipation. High-fiber diets and stool softeners can reduce the likelihood of constipation following the surgery.

6. You may shower after surgery whenever you wish. Remove the surgical garment and dressings. After showering, pat the incision areas gently with a towel. Reapply Polysporin Ointment and a clean cotton dressing.

7. Keep your surgical garment clean. It is machine washable and dryable. It's a good idea to have two surgical garments so you can wear one while the other is being laundered. Bicycle pants work very nicely as an alternative corset.

8. No driving until pain medication has worn off.

9. One week post-op you can do some walking, but nothing strenuous for at least four weeks after surgery.

10. If any activity hurts, *stop it.*

11. Take a multivitamin and iron supplement following surgery. Be sure to discuss your dosage with your doctor before medicating (it depends on your blood loss).

Supplies to have at home: Polysporin Ointment, two-by-two-inch cotton gauze squares and paper bandage tape.

THE RECOVERY PERIOD

You're going to feel unbelievably sore for about three to six days, as if someone had given you a severe beating. Then the situation becomes tolerably uncomfortable for another couple of weeks, until finally it passes. Take your prescription pain medication provided by the office. Why suffer through those first few days more than necessary? By the end of the first week you can probably switch over to Tylenol and make do on that until the discomfort disappears.

Bruising is normal and will usually begin to subside two to four weeks after surgery. Homeopathic doses of Arnica (as described on page 21) will greatly help to reduce the bruising and soreness.

Swelling is common following liposuction and has been known to last for several weeks. The surgical girdle will help control abdominal swelling. Leg and ankle swelling can be improved by elevating the legs as often as possible. Also, try to maintain a low-salt diet to discourage water retention.

Initially there will be irregularity, lumpiness and multiple areas of bruising. Your doctor may recommend physical therapy with ultrasound and massage for two to three weeks. This smoothes the irregularities and speeds healing.

Don't attempt light exercise or any aerobics until four to six weeks post-op, and that time period will depend on your individual bruising and swelling. If you have any bruises left, check with your doctor before lifting a leg in exercise. Then you can gently and slowly work your way back up to a normal exercise level. A good rule is, if it hurts, *don't do it.*

If you're dieting, don't start any extreme starvation programs until three weeks post-op. For proper healing purposes you really do need to maintain a healthy and balanced diet those two to three weeks following surgery.

Do not become depressed if you don't suddenly see a dramatic change in your body the first few days after surgery. Swelling and scar tissue can disguise your final results, which should become apparent 6 to 12 weeks post-op.

PROBLEM SIGNS

Medical problems during the post-liposuction healing process are rare, but you should keep an eye on the incision lines for any possible infection. As with any surgery, there is a possibility of internal bleeding, and at the first sign of a raised and sore area or an unusual bruise you should call your doctor.

Other long-term problems from liposuction could include cellulite conditions appearing worse; areas of wrinkling or rippled and uneven skin; and lumpy, uneven results that could cause silhouette irregularities.

Incidentally, many liposuction cases will need some small touch-up surgery to make things look great.

MAKEUP TRICKS

You can apply makeup to camouflage bruising 48 hours after the sutures have been removed, and only if the incision lines are completely healed over and dry. Dermablend, Physicians Formula Velvet Film, Max Factor Pan Stick, Clinique Continuous Coverage, Prescriptives Camouflage Creme, Cover Mark or Natural Cover are all very effective products.

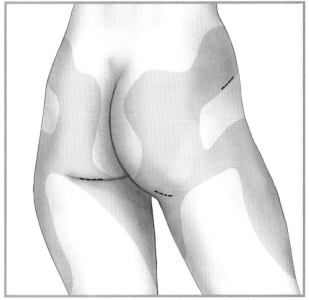

Small incisions are made for entrance of the suctioning tube. The shaded space indicates the areas to be liposuctioned.

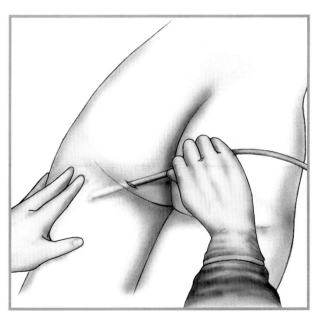

The tube is inserted and the surgeon manipulates the tube in between the skin and the muscle, removing the fat from the area.

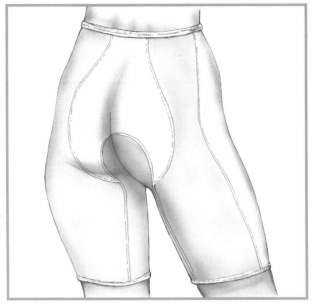

A surgical girdle that you will wear 24 hours a day for a minimum of seven days (or longer according to your doctor's instructions) will help reduce swelling.

CHAPTER SIXTEEN

Abdominoplasty

(TUMMY TUCK)

• • •

APPROXIMATE COST:$3,700–$6,000

There may be additional charges for surgical facilities and anesthesia. Be sure to request this information.

APPROXIMATE TIME UNTIL COMPLETELY HEALED:

You'll be happy with the initial results immediately. You'll probably look good three months post-op. It takes a full year, however, for everything to be completely healed and normal.

BEFORE YOU SET A DATE

There is a deep fat pad lying below the belly button that is physically exclusive to women (men develop a "spare tire" around the middle of their body instead). Also, after several pregnancies many women develop wrinkled and hanging abdominal skin, particularly if an abdominal hernia has occurred. If you want to eliminate these conditions, liposuction will not be enough to do the trick. You will need to have an abdominoplasty, commonly known as a tummy tuck.

Like liposuction, a tummy tuck is not an alternative to weight reduction. It will improve your abdominal silhouette by surgically giving you a smoother and flatter stomach. However, if you gain a lot of weight your stomach will once again expand.

The trade-off with a tummy tuck is a flatter, smoother stomach versus a rather conspicuous permanent scar. Depending on the amount of skin to be removed, the scar can be anything from a small incision to a long line running from one hip across the pubic area and up to the other hip. So before you decide on surgery, be very aware of the trade-off; you'll have a flatter and unwrinkled tummy that will look great in a one-piece bathing suit, but buck naked you will be left with an obvious scar.

Unlike liposuction, abdominoplasty is a serious operation. Often the patient must give a pint of his or her own blood before surgery in case blood loss occurs.

If a patient is suffering from a massive apron of fat (such as after a huge weight loss) a panniculectomy is performed. Symptoms relevant to this surgery include a breakdown of the abdominal muscle structure, strain on the lumbar spine, chronic low-back pain and difficulty in walking. This procedure is definitely more therapeutic than cosmetic in nature. If you feel you require a panniculectomy, discuss it in great detail with your internist as well as a plastic surgeon.

PRESURGICAL INSTRUCTIONS

- You will be given blood and lab tests approximately two weeks prior to surgery. Take no aspirin or aspirin-containing products for two weeks prior to your surgery and 10 days after (see list of medications to avoid). You may take Tylenol.

- If you take medication daily, notify your doctor. Also inform him if you develop an illness or cold within a week of your surgery.

- If you're a smoker you should clearly understand that nicotine can impair and delay healing. Most offices will suggest quitting a week to 10 days before surgery, a week post-op. If it were me, I'd stop smoking a minimum of three weeks prior to surgery and not touch a cigarette for a full month post-op. Who needs to be left with scars worse than normal and other complications as a result of smoking through the pre- and postsurgical period?

THE DAY BEFORE SURGERY

Do not eat or drink anything after midnight.

THE DAY OF SURGERY

- You may rinse and brush your teeth, but *do not eat or drink anything*. Some doctor's offices may ask you to take pills with a small amount of water the day of surgery.

- Wear no makeup and remove your contact lenses and dentures for surgery. *Do not put any moisturizer on your eyes or face.*

- Do not bring any jewelry or valuables. Wear a robe, housecoat or warmup suit that buttons or zips in the front and flat shoes. *No tight-fitting clothes.*

- *Someone must drive you home and spend the first night with you.*

- Postoperative instructions regarding activity, medications and office visits will be given following your surgery.

THE SURGERY

Abdominoplasty surgery takes approximately three to four hours. Add an additional half hour for preparation and anesthesia. There are normally four people in the operating room with you: the surgeon, the anesthesiologist and two surgical nurses. You will be given antibiotics through your I.V. during surgery. Because this is considered major surgery, the doctor may choose to have an assistant present and the procedure may take place in the hospital rather than in the office surgical facilities.

Unlike liposuction, abdominoplasty is a rather extensive procedure. An incision is made from under one hip bone, down under the low abdominal crease across the pubic area and up to the other hip bone. An incision may also be made around the umbilicus (belly button).

The skin is freed-up (separated) from the abdominal incision line clear up to the rib cage area under the breasts. The abdominal fat pad is surgically removed, and if hernia repair is necessary (which is quite common), the surgeon tightens the loose underlying tissue and two muscles together with sutures. This procedure will diminish the size of the waistline to a certain degree, but don't look for an hourglass waistline post-op—it just won't happen.

The freed-up skin is brought downward, and the surgeon cuts a new opening for the belly button that is then sutured closed around the navel.

The excess skin is trimmed away to fit the abdominal incision, and two drains are inserted into the abdominal area for a couple of days to prevent bleeding problems. The abdominal incision is immediately closed with sutures that will be removed in 14 days. Steri-strips or staples may also reinforce the sutured incision line. A firm elastic binder is applied to the entire area clear up to the rib cage.

POSTSURGICAL INSTRUCTIONS

1. Physical activity should be limited to movements that are comfortable. For the first two days you should stay reclined with bent knees, getting up only to go to the bathroom. Stay close to home the first two weeks after surgery.

2. Wear the supportive garment that was selected prior to the surgery 24 hours a day for four to six weeks. As a general rule, the supportive garment should be worn until the bruising and discomfort have subsided.

3. Polysporin Ointment should be applied to the sutures daily until suture removal (approximately seven days). Use a cotton-tipped applicator to apply the ointment.

4. Continue the antibiotics as instructed. If you develop diarrhea, discontinue the antibiotics and notify your doctor.

5. Anesthetics and pain medication tend to produce constipation. High-fiber diets and stool softeners will help reduce the likelihood of constipation following surgery.

6. You may shower after surgery whenever you wish. Remove the surgical garment and dressings. After showering, pat the incision areas gently with a towel. Reapply Polysporin Ointment and a clean cotton dressing.

7. Keep your surgical garment clean. It is machine washable and dryable. It's a good idea to have two surgical garments so you can wear one while the other is being laundered. Bicycle pants work very nicely as an alternative corset.

8. No driving until pain medication has worn off.

9. Take a multivitamin and an iron supplement following surgery. Be sure to discuss your dosage with your doctor before medicating (it depends on your blood loss).

10. No exercise or aerobics for six to eight weeks post-op.

Supplies to have at home: Polysporin Ointment, two-by-two-inch cotton gauze squares and paper bandage tape.

THE RECOVERY PERIOD

Because abdominoplasty is major surgery, you should expect to feel rather weak for several weeks post-op. It usually takes at least eight full weeks to recover your normal energy and stamina. Don't be surprised if you experience some depression for a few days after surgery. It's a common reaction, and it will pass as you regain your strength.

Be prepared for some serious discomfort following this surgery. You will need to remain in a sitting position the first two to four days. In other words, even when you lie down or stand up, your knees must remain bent at all times. If you straighten up, you'll rip out your stitches! The first couple of weeks are really tough, and you'll need to take some prescribed pain medication during this period and perhaps even a little longer.

Because everything has been pulled down and repositioned so tightly, you will not be physically able to stand up straight for about two weeks after the operation. For goodness sake, don't fight it and attempt to straighten up too soon. Many patients develop temporary lower-back problems as a result of having to stay bent all this time, but the back problems usually clear up once they're walking normally again. Low-back exercises are frequently helpful, but only after six to eight weeks post-op and with your doctor's permission.

Prepare yourself for some serious swelling and bruising for several weeks; wearing your surgical girdle religiously will help control the swelling.

Another temporary problem that often develops is a sloughing of the skin in the area. This condition clears up as the area begins to calm down through more progressed healing, usually after the fourth week post-op. Actually, you'll see some skin sloughing around most all surgical incision lines, whether they've been pulled tight or not. It all goes away.

Don't become depressed if the abdominal scar looks thick and puffy. The scar will flatten out in 6 to 12 months, and many people opt for a little liposuction to reduce any remaining fullness around the healed incision. Sometimes an unacceptable scar will remain, and you'll want to have a scar revision at a later date. Scar revision surgery is reasonably uncomplicated, and a knowledgeable and careful surgeon can accomplish major improvements with this procedure.

If you're dieting, don't start any extreme programs until at least three weeks after surgery. For proper healing purposes you need to maintain a healthy and balanced diet those first few post-op weeks.

You can usually return to work (depending on the extent and severity of the surgery) three to four weeks after the procedure.

Absolutely no exercise or aerobics until six to eight weeks post-op, and only with your doctor's permission.

PROBLEM SIGNS

If there is any sign of infection, call your doctor at once. Raised, sore areas and uneven (one-sided) swelling are symptoms that could indicate internal bleeding, and your doctor must be informed immediately.

Any buildup of fluid in the abdominal area is a serious problem that your doctor will need to know about right away. The area will be swollen and you will actually be able to feel water in there. Your doctor will surgically drain the fluid out of the area as soon as possible.

MAKEUP TRICKS

You can apply makeup to camouflage bruising 48 hours after the sutures have been removed, but only if the incision lines are completely healed over and dry. Dermablend, Physicians Formula Velvet Film, Max Factor Pan Stick, Clinique Continuous Coverage, Prescriptives Camouflage Creme, Cover Mark or Natural Cover all are very effective products. The makeup creams will not camouflage the abdominal scar but will cover up any redness or discoloration of it.

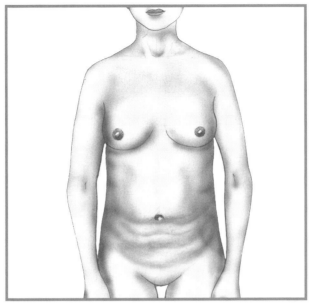

Folds and enlarged layers of loose skin are often the chief complaint of a patient seeking abdominoplasty.

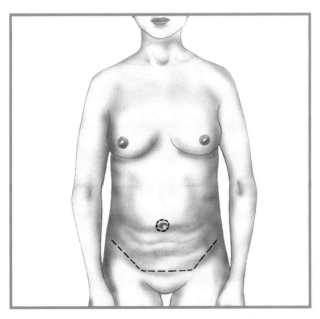

An incision is made from under one hip bone, down under the lower abdominal crease across the pubic area and up to the other hip bone. An incision is also made around the umbilicus (belly button).

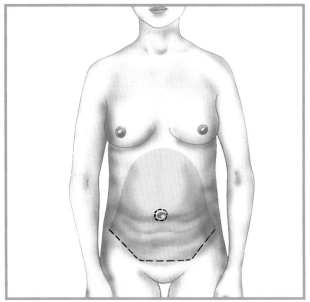

The skin is freed up from the abdominal incision line clear up to the rib cage area under the breasts (as shown by the shaded area), and the fat pad is removed.

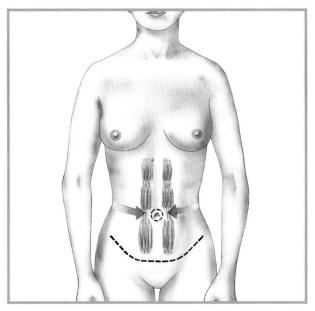

If hernia repair is necessary, the surgeon will tighten the loose underlying tissue and two muscles together with sutures.

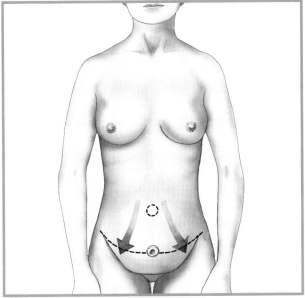

The freed-up skin is brought downward and a new opening is cut for the belly button, which is sutured closed around the navel.

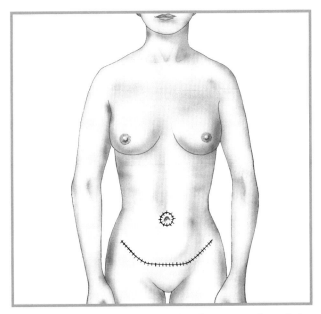

The freed-up skin is brought downward and the excess skin trimmed away before suturing.

ABDOMINOPLASTY

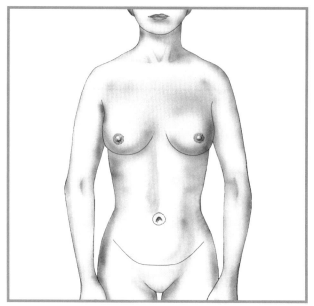

Post-surgery leaves you with a flatter, smoother tummy. The incision line leaves a permanent scar.

CHAPTER SEVENTEEN

Cheek, Chin, Pectoral and Calf Implants

• • •

CHEEK IMPLANTS / APPROXIMATE COST: $2,500–$4,500

There may be additional charges for surgical facilities and anesthesia. Be sure to request this information.

APPROXIMATE TIME UNTIL COMPLETELY HEALED:

Three months.

BEFORE YOU SET A DATE

Prior to surgery, be sure you and your doctor have clearly decided upon the actual size of the cheek implant and the end results you expect to accomplish by reshaping the face with the implants. Too often people wake up from this particular procedure quite horrified to discover a distortion in their face they never expected, usually as a result of implants that are simply too large.

One of the biggest risks of cheek implant surgery is not medical; it's being dissatisfied with the end result. Cheek implants produce an extremely dramatic and rather severe change to the face that can be difficult to imagine accurately.

The correct question to ask yourself presurgery is, "Do I want more prominent cheekbones?" If you're expecting to fill in a fallen face or plump out facial lines with cheek implants, forget it. That's not what they're for. If you put cheek implants into your face, it will accomplish only one thing: you'll have more defined cheekbones. Once you understand this, the most important decision you must make concerns the size of the implant. You'd be wise to insist on the most subtle implant that would be appropriate for your face. Nothing looks more distorted and terrible than cheek implants that aren't subtle. (Incidentally, implants known as submalar implants are available for the purpose of filling in fallen or sunken cheeks. However, they tend to look unnatural—like a bad case of mumps— and are a separate subject and procedure, not to be confused with malar cheek implants, which we are discussing here.)

PRESURGICAL INSTRUCTIONS

- You will be given blood and lab tests approximately two weeks prior to your surgery. Take no aspirin or aspirin-containing products, as they can cause bleeding and bruising. (See list of medications to avoid for two weeks prior to your surgery and one week after.) You may take Tylenol.

- If you take medication daily, notify your doctor. Also tell him if you develop an illness, cold or any skin infections within a week of your surgery.

THE DAY BEFORE SURGERY

Do not eat or drink anything after midnight.

THE DAY OF SURGERY

- You may rinse and brush your teeth, but *do not eat or drink anything*. Some offices may ask you to take pills with a small amount of water the day of surgery.

- Do not bring any jewelry or valuables. Wear a robe, housecoat or warmup suit that buttons or zips in the front, and wear flat shoes. *No tight-fitting clothes.*

- *Someone must drive you home and stay with you the first night.*

- Postoperative instructions regarding activity, medications and office visits will be given following your surgery.

THE SURGERY

Cheek implant surgery takes approximately an hour to an hour and a half. Add an additional half hour for preparation and anesthesia. There are normally four people in the operating room with you: the surgeon, the anesthesiologist and two surgical nurses. You will be given general anesthesia intravenously. An I.V. antibiotic will also be administered.

An incision is made inside the mouth as high up toward the cheekbone as possible. Occasionally the incision is made in the lower eyelid or hairline area. The implant is inserted through the incision and placed over your own cheekbone. The incision line is closed with dissolving stitches.

The biggest risk of this procedure is that the patient can be left with numbness above the upper lip as a result of pressure the implant places on the infraorbital nerve (the nerve running from the eye down the cheek to the mouth). Usually this numbness goes away in two to three months. If the implant is too large, the numbness will remain, indicating that mechanical damage has occurred. A good doctor is always very careful to avoid causing permanent nerve damage during this procedure, but be aware that it is a possibility.

POSTSURGICAL INSTRUCTIONS

1. Rest quietly for one or two days. Then limit yourself to light activities for at least two weeks.

2. Avoid straining, exercise or head-down positions, all of which can cause unnecessary swelling or bleeding.

3. Keep on a liquid diet (nothing extremely hot!) for the first 24 hours post-op. Then stay on a soft-food diet until you feel comfortable enough to return to your normal diet.

4. *Do not brush your teeth* until the fourth day post-op. Just gently rinse with salt and warm water or Hydrogel.

THE RECOVERY PERIOD

Expect some swelling and bruising after surgery. The bruising usually disappears within two weeks; You'll be able to begin to judge your finished results in approximately two to four weeks. Expect some tenderness for a couple of weeks, and possibly the numbness above the upper lip, as was previously described.

PROBLEM SIGNS

If you have constant severe pain or any fever or indication of infection, call the doctor immediately.

Uneven swelling could be an indication of bleeding or (more unlikely) that the implant has slipped and will require quick repositioning. If the implant has not been correctly placed, it can slip downward toward the mouth inside the cheek. It can also rotate, causing the lower lid of the eye to pull down. These are both rare occurrences. Don't panic; just get to your doctor right away so he can make the necessary surgical adjustments.

MAKEUP TRICKS

You can cover temporary bruising with the appropriate color of Dermablend, Physicians Formula Velvet Film, Max Factor Pan Stick, Clinique Continuous Coverage, Prescriptives Camouflage Creme, Cover Mark or Natural Cover.

CHIN IMPLANTS / APPROXIMATE COST: $2,700–$3,200

There may be additional charges for surgical facilities and anesthesia. Be sure to request this information.

APPROXIMATE TIME UNTIL COMPLETELY HEALED:

Four to six weeks.

BEFORE YOU SET A DATE

Chin implants are one of the most common implant procedures. Prior to surgery, be sure you and your doctor have determined the appropriate size implant for your face. The implant obviously will have to balance and blend with the proportions of your nose and your facial structure. An implant that's too large will look really dreadful, so carefully discuss the size decision with your doctor before the surgery.

PRESURGICAL INSTRUCTIONS

- You will be given blood and lab tests approximately two weeks prior to your surgery. Take no aspirin or aspirin-containing products; they can cause bleeding and bruising. (See list of medications to avoid for two weeks prior to your surgery and one week after.) You may take Tylenol.
- If you take medication daily, notify your doctor. Also inform him if you develop an illness, cold or any skin infections within a week of your surgery.
- If you're a smoker you should clearly understand that nicotine can impair and delay healing. Most offices will suggest quitting a week to 10 days before surgery, a week post-op. If it were me, I'd stop smoking a minimum of three weeks prior to surgery and not touch a cigarette for a full month post-op. Who needs to be left with scars worse than normal and other complications as a result of smoking through the pre- and postsurgical period?

THE DAY BEFORE SURGERY

Do not eat or drink anything after midnight.

THE DAY OF SURGERY

- You may rinse and brush your teeth, but *do not eat or drink anything*. Some offices may ask you to take pills with a small amount of water the day of surgery.

- Do not bring any jewelry or valuables. Wear a robe, housecoat or warmup suit that buttons or zips in the front, and wear flat shoes. *No tight-fitting clothes.*

- *Someone must drive you home and stay with you the first night.*

- Postoperative instructions regarding activity, medications and office visits will be given following your surgery.

THE SURGERY

Chin implant surgery takes approximately one half hour. Add an additional half hour for preparation and anesthesia. There are normally four people in the operating room with you: the surgeon, the anesthesiologist and two surgical nurses. The procedure can be done under a general anesthetic or with an I.V. sedation combined with injections of local anesthesia into the chin area.

The chin implant is made of Silastic rubber. An incision is made either inside the mouth down in the area between the gums and chin region or under the chin. The implant is inserted down through the incision, against the bone between the two nerves that run along either side of the jaw. Unlike cheek implants, the risk of nerve damage with chin implants is very low.

The incision is closed with dissolving stitches or in the mouth with nylon sutures under the chin. Tape is placed over the chin and under the jaw to support the implant for five to seven days.

POSTSURGICAL INSTRUCTIONS

1. Rest quietly for one or two days. Then limit yourself to light activities for at least two weeks.

2. Avoid straining, exercise or head-down positions, all of which can cause unnecessary swelling or bleeding.

3. Keep on a liquid diet (nothing extremely hot!) for the first 24 hours post-op. Then stay on a soft-food diet until you feel comfortable enough to return to your normal diet.

4. *Do not brush your teeth* until the fourth day after surgery. Just gently rinse with salt and warm water or Hydrogel.

5. Avoid excessive talking the first 24 hours. Too much talking can cause greater-than-normal swelling.

THE RECOVERY PERIOD

Expect some swelling and bruising. The bruising will disappear in a couple of weeks. The swelling can last as long as two to three months. The worst thing about a chin implant is the initial discomfort, because the two chin nerves have literally been pulled apart to house the implant. Expect to wake up feeling incredibly sore and tender for the first few days. A less severe tenderness will last for another four to six weeks until it completely normalizes.

PROBLEM SIGNS

If you have severe constant pain (more intense than what you've been prepared for), call your doctor. Any uneven swelling could be an indication of bleeding or the unlikely possibility that the implant has slipped and may require surgical repositioning. If there is any fever or indication of infection, call your doctor immediately.

MAKEUP TRICKS

You can cover temporary bruising with the appropriate color of Dermablend, Physicians Formula Velvet Film, Max Factor Pan Stick, Clinique Continuous Coverage, Cover Mark, Prescriptives Camouflage Creme, Cover Mark or Natural Cover.

PECTORAL AND CALF IMPLANTS

Some men are having pectoral implants to enlarge their chest size. The implants are custom-made and can feel quite unnatural and hard to the touch under the skin.

Calf implants are also available to add shape to the lower leg. The downside to calf implants is the visible scars left on the leg.

Both pectoral and calf-implant surgeries are relatively new procedures, and most doctors are still quite skeptical about them. If you insist on pursuing these particular implants, I urge you to go very slowly and carefully.

Because there's such a lack of data regarding these two implants, I prefer to close the subject here and advise you to personally question your doctors.

CHEEK IMPLANTS

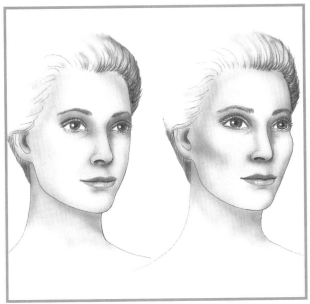

Before and after cheeks. A cheek implant can pro-vide a beautiful and subtle contour to the area.

CHIN IMPLANT

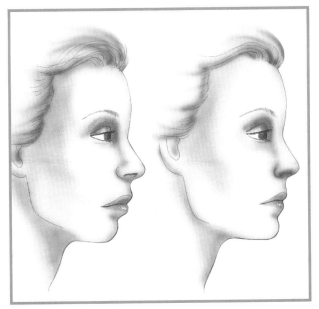

Before and after chin. Chin implants can imme-diately and dramatically provide appropriate balance to the entire face.

CALF IMPLANTS

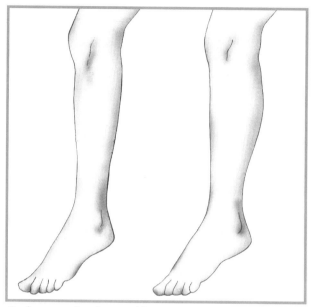

Before and after calf. Exceptionally shapeless calves could be improved with a subtle implant.

CHAPTER EIGHTEEN

Light and Medium Facial Peels

• • •

LIGHT PEELS: GLYCOLIC (FRUIT) ACID PEELS / APPROXIMATE COST: $200–$300 *per session*

A minimum of two or three sessions, a month apart, are usually recommended. The end results of glycolic acid peels are cumulative, and some plastic surgeons and dermatologists recommend a series of up to six peels to achieve desired results.

APPROXIMATE TIME UNTIL NORMAL BETWEEN PEELS:

One week.

BEFORE YOU SET A DATE

Glycolic acid is a light peel that will improve the overall quality of the skin. Most uneven skin discolorations will benefit from the series, and the overall texture of the skin will be smoother and fresher. Tiny fine lines can be refined with glycolic acid. However, elimination of moderate lines requires a medium peel (trichloroacetic acid) and deep lines and wrinkles necessitate a phenol peel.

PREPROCEDURE INSTRUCTIONS

If you have a history of facial or lip herpes (cold sores), have your doctor place you on five Zovirax capsules a day for one day prior to each peel and five days afterward. Some doctors place you on Zovirax the day before the procedure and for 10 days thereafter. Listen to your doctor! If you break out in herpes during any of the peel recovery, you could be left with permanent scarring, and you need to avoid this at all costs by medicating with Zovirax.

Apart from this premedication, no other preparation is necessary. The peels are usually done as an outpatient procedure in the doctor's office. No medication is generally necessary for glycolic acid peels, so you can take your usual medication if you're on any daily program.

THE PROCEDURE

The skin is usually cleaned with soap and water; sometimes acetone is applied to "degrease" the surface.

The actual peel takes only 15 to 30 minutes. The glycolic acid is applied with cotton balls or swabs and is usually a concentration of 50 percent to 70 percent strength. The acid is applied in sections. Usually each cheek is done separately; the forehead, chin and mouth areas are also done as separate units. This technique applies to all peels.

The glycolic acid solution is left on the skin anywhere from 3 to 6 minutes. You will experience mild burning and redness of the skin. Sometimes the skin will "frost"—a white film will appear on its surface. After 3 to 6 minutes, depending on your skin's reaction, the glycolic acid is neutralized with ice water compresses that are left on for 5 to 10 minutes. The instant the ice water hits your skin you're out of any real discomfort, and the mild burning usually subsides after 15 minutes.

You'll have some redness and some mild swelling of the face, but nothing really terrible. In fact, you should feel absolutely fine. Because there was no premedication, you could even return to work.

POSTPROCEDURE INSTRUCTIONS

Gently cleanse your skin. *Avoid any abrasive products.* Avoid sun exposure during the healing period.

THE RECOVERY PERIOD

During the first week post-peel, you will experience some peeling of the skin in varying degrees depending on your skin type. It could be a mild to minimal peeling, or a more significant peeling of the skin, similar to a severe sunburn. The peeling is treated with mild emollients or moisturizers.

PROBLEM SIGNS

The peeling usually stops three to seven days following the procedure. Although there are no side effects to the peel, you could have some postinflammatory hyperpigmentation (redness). If this occurs, call your doctor for instructions.

MAKEUP TRICKS

Moisturize generously following the peel. You can apply your normal makeup three to seven days after the procedure, depending on when your skin sloughing has stopped.

In between the series of glycolic acid peels, you are usually advised to use a cleanser or moisturizer containing glycolic acid at home.

MEDIUM PEELS: TRICHLOROACETIC ACID (TCA) PEELS / APPROXIMATE COST: $1,200–$2,000

APPROXIMATE TIME UNTIL COMPLETELY HEALED:

10 days.

BEFORE YOU SET A DATE

Trichloroacetic (TCA) peels are quite effective in correcting sun-damaged skin and improving skin that has suffered the natural aging process. TCA peels, however, will not remove deep aging lines. Some growths and pre-skin cancers are also effectively treated by TCA.

Meet with your doctor before the procedure to decide which areas should be treated. With a TCA or phenol peel I recommend a full-face peel because the skin tone will not match the rest of your face if you only "spot peel," and you'll need to constantly wear makeup in order to blend your skin tones.

Glycolic acid peels and TCA peels are quite different. A glycolic acid peel is light and superficial, almost like a deep facial. A TCA peel is a serious peel that requires a good week to 10 days of recovery and hiding out at home while the healing process goes through its various stages.

PREPROCEDURE INSTRUCTIONS

- You can take your normal medication up until the time of the procedure, but because you will be given sedation, *you must tell your doctor every single medication you have swallowed! Don't forget to report a single pill!*

- You can eat a light breakfast the morning of the procedure.

- Because you will be given preoperative sedation, you will not be allowed to drive, so arrange to have someone bring you to the office and pick you up about two or three hours later.

You will not require hospitalization or an aftercare facility following a TCA procedure; you'll recover nicely at home. A conscientious doctor will call you and monitor your progress the first three days following the procedure.

- Some doctors will place you on several weeks of Retin-A before your TCA peel. Other doctors feel this preconditioning of the skin is unnecessary.

- It is imperative that you medicate with Zovirax capsules five times a day prior to the procedure and 10 days post-procedure to prevent facial herpes.

THE DAY BEFORE THE PROCEDURE

Shampoo your hair the night before your peel, as you won't be able to shampoo for several days following the procedure.

THE DAY OF THE PROCEDURE

Come to the office with no makeup on your face, and wear a shirt that can be unbuttoned. Some doctors prescribe Valium to be taken prior to the procedure.

THE PROCEDURE

The peel will take anywhere from one to two hours. Add an additional half hour preparation time.

You will arrive at the office premedicated, having taken Valium orally, and you will be given an injection or I.V. of Demerol and Vistaril to suppress any pain.

Skin preparation for the TCA solution is then applied: either acetone, Jessners solution or carbon dioxide in block form.

The skin is now ready to receive the TCA. Various concentrations of TCA can be applied, from 20 percent to 50 percent, depending upon the depth of the peel. The stronger the TCA, the deeper the peel, and that will be determined by the specific areas of the face as well as the amount of damage to be corrected. For instance, a lower percent solution is used on the delicate skin under the eyes, while a higher percent TCA would be used over the upper lip area.

As with all peels, the TCA is applied with a cotton swab, and the face is done in sections. Make absolutely sure your doctor feathers the TCA solution under your jaw bone and chin so that you won't have a line of demarcation between your face and your jaw. The doctor must mark the line while you're sitting up just prior to surgery. He will swab the section of skin until an even frosting is achieved. The process is as follows: application of TCA, followed by a burning of the skin that turns pink and then white into a frost. The whiteness of the frost disappears in 15 or 20 minutes, leaving the skin slightly swollen and bright pink, like a bad sunburn.

As the TCA is applied to each section, expect it to burn quite a bit (it's bad but not intolerable). Once an area is completed, ice is applied to that area to counteract the burning. The ice does kill the burning sensation within seconds of contact with the skin, so just grit your teeth and know that the discomfort will be over as soon as you're iced.

POSTPROCEDURE INSTRUCTIONS

The most important postsurgical instruction is to keep your head elevated to reduce the swelling. When you go home, sit up as much as possible. If you're lying down, prop your head up with three or four pillows and continue this for at least four days. The effects of swelling are temporary and usually last three or four days.

Do not shampoo your hair for at least four or five days. You want your skin to harden, so the steam from shampooing is a bad idea. Do not wash your face; instead apply ice water compresses or cool spritzes with water.

Eat normally. No exercise until all your swelling is completely gone (approximately two weeks following the procedure), and be prepared to hide out at home for a good week.

Apply antibiotic ointment after your skin has turned brown, usually three or four days post-procedure. Continue the ointment until your face has completely peeled.

THE RECOVERY PERIOD

You really won't be in any significant pain. The real discomfort was experienced during application of the TCA solution. Once you're home, you'll feel a tight sensation over the skin. Expect to swell up more than you thought, but do call your doctor at once if the swelling becomes excessive. If necessary, your doctor can prescribe medication to reduce the swelling.

After the swelling subsides, the skin, which is usually a reddish to a dusty brown color, will start to turn a chocolate brown. Once the skin turns brown, the patient should start using a topical antibiotic ointment such as Polysporin or Bacitracin. Usually products with Neomycin or Neosporin are not recommended because they have a history of allergic reactions. In general, antibiotic ointments and creams should not be used longer than three days postop as they also have a tendency to produce irritation. Your goal is to keep the brown skin constantly moist as it peels.

If you get cabin fever staying home while the brown skin is peeling away, you can continue to apply the ointment and leave the house. But be prepared to scare small children and to explain why you look so creepy.

The peeling process usually takes about 7 to 10 days. Once the brown skin is peeling, it's best to allow it to come off naturally. Don't pick, or you'll end up with an uneven skin tone and possibly some scarring.

After the brown skin has peeled off, your skin will have a beautiful pink glow. A sunscreen should be used for at least six months to protect this new skin from ultraviolet light. Wait at least 48 hours after the brown skin has peeled off before applying any sunscreen, and if your new skin still seems sensitive to it, wait a few days longer.

PROBLEM SIGNS

TCA peels are usually a safe and effective procedure, but complications could include discoloration—either a lightening or darkening of the skin in some areas.

The best candidates for peels are fair-complexioned people with blond hair and blue eyes. Olive-skinned people with dark eyes have a higher risk of problems. A test is usually done before the procedure along the forehead hairline to make sure that the patient has normal healing from TCA and there are no pigmentary changes.

The chances of scarring are minimal, but it can happen, especially if higher concentrations of the chemical are used. In these cases the cheekbones and the jaw line are highly susceptible to scarring.

Because of the use of the greasy antibiotic ointment, be prepared for a possible outbreak of acne after the procedure.

Before and after the peel, most offices are recommending the use of bleaching agents. The bleaching agent, which is generally hydroquinone, is combined with Retin-A or glycolic acid. The bleach will help prevent dark spots. Retin-A or glycolic acid used preoperatively will speed recovery.

MAKEUP TRICKS

After your brown skin has completely peeled, moisturize your new skin for two days. Then you can moisturize and apply your normal makeup.

CHAPTER NINETEEN

Deep Peels: The Phenol Peel

• • •

APPROXIMATE COST: $2,500–$5,500

There may be additional charges for surgical facilities and anesthesia. Be sure to request this information.

APPROXIMATE TIME UNTIL COMPLETELY HEALED:

Two weeks, not including the six to eight weeks it will take for the pinkness to fade.

BEFORE YOU SET A DATE

A deep phenol peel will remove the majority of lines and wrinkles from your face, clarify extreme discoloration and smooth out acne pits. It also tightens the skin. This procedure is rarely performed on someone under 35 years of age unless there's excessive sun damage.

The results from a deep phenol peel are quite dramatic, but do not confuse this procedure with a face-lift: the two surgeries produce completely different results. A phenol peel will give you smooth, even-toned, wrinkle-free skin. A face-lift tightens and lifts up the sagging areas of your face and neck. Both procedures are considered major surgery as they both require general anesthesia and surgical monitoring.

The biggest trade-off to doing a deep phenol peel is that you will be left with a permanent loss of pigment in the face. The skin becomes extremely white. You will have a wrinkle-free face, but you'll have to constantly wear a makeup foundation that ensures your face will match your neck and body. Depending on your lifestyle, it might not be a huge price to pay if you dream of being wrinkle-free.

You will be required to have a complete physical workup, including an AIDS test. A deep phenol peel is serious business, and it's imperative that the patient is in top health. Phenol acts as a drug: it enters the bloodstream and the tissue. If an excessive concentration is allowed to build up, it can be damaging. Your internist must also test you for kidney function, since the kidneys are primarily responsible for phenol clearance. Phenol peeling is NOT recommended for people with kidney problems. Pregnant women should not have a phenol peel. Phenol clearance also is why the doctor will apply this acid solution to your face one section at a time and wait between each application. This gives the solution time to clear your system as you proceed with the acid application.

One of the most important conversations you must have before phenol surgery is with your doctor's anesthesiologist. Phenol peeling penetrates the skin deeply, and the key to your comfort during those very raw 48 hours after waking up lies with the anesthesiologist. Some drugs included in the anesthesia will leave you in a state of seminumbness, especially for the first 12 hours upon awakening (usually the worst time for experiencing pain). Believe me, you'll want to float through that first day or two following the surgery. Most people (not everyone, however) say it could be a rough and painful couple of days without the appropriate drugs. Pain medication will also be given orally as needed.

If you are not allowed to take painkillers, I would seriously reconsider having a phenol peel. Getting through the first and perhaps second day without drugs could be extremely painful.

It is imperative that you medicate with Zovirax before surgery and 10 days through the recovery period. Don't skip a single pill, because a breakout of herpes could leave you with deep and unsightly scarring.

Another subject you should discuss with your surgeon is

whether you want him to delicately "feather" the phenol peel under your jaw line and chin so that you won't be left with a color line at your jaw. The doctor must mark this line while you're sitting up just prior to surgery.

PRESURGICAL INSTRUCTIONS

No sunbathing is allowed before surgery. No food or liquids are allowed after midnight the night before surgery. You can continue to smoke if you insist, but remember that smoking does slow down the healing process to a large degree.

THE DAY OF SURGERY

Arrive at the office or hospital with no makeup on your face. Wear a shirt that buttons down the front, or loose clothes that unzip down the front.

THE SURGERY

The entire procedure takes two to three hours. Add a half hour for preparation and anesthesia. The skin is prepared with acetone, Jessners solution or carbon dioxide in block form.

The phenol acid is applied section by section, with time in between to allow the acid to clear from the system. The skin frosts, turns waxen and then becomes a deep brownish red. Actually, the skin blisters (as with a severe burn) and forms this brownish-red crust.

Bandages are applied to the facial areas that are in need of deeper treatment and are left on 24 to 48 hours following the procedure. Brief anesthesia is required to remove the bandages at the appropriate time.

The neck should not be peeled with phenol acid, as it can create serious scarring there.

POSTSURGICAL INSTRUCTIONS

Plan to stay home and hide for a week to 10 days. You are going to be ugly beyond belief the first six or seven days after surgery.

For the first 48 hours, simply rest and keep activity to a minimum. Your doctor will check you the day after the peel. It's advisable to spend the first night and preferably the second night in an aftercare facility. After all, you've had general anesthesia and a considerable shock to the system. You'll also need to be on a special high-protein liquid diet, and you must try not to speak during that first day post-op. It's best to be monitored by professionals. By the third day post-op, your bandages have been removed during your office visit. The skin will look raw. *Don't panic*; it's normal at this point. Now you will begin to spread your antibiotic ointment all over the face. Apply the ointment several times during the day. The most important factor is the necessity to always keep a soft crust on the face. The continual application of ointment prevents the crust from turning into a hard scab, which is something you want to avoid at all costs. Skin always heals best when it's coated and soft.

The fourth day post-op you can gently wash your face four to six times a day with Ivory soap; reapply the antibiotic ointment to the entire face after each washing.

Prepare yourself. You are going to look quite hideous from the second through the sixth day after surgery. The skin "weeps" continually during this period, so between the weeping, the ointment and a face full of brownish-red soft skin, you're not going to want to do much besides washing and greasing your face and hiding out.

By the seventh day post-op, most of the brownish-red skin is off and the weeping has stopped. Your fresh skin will be smooth and reddish pink in color, like a sunburn. Wait at least 48 hours before applying any makeup. Skin-care products such as cleansing lotions, softening oils and sunscreens should be prescribed or provided to you by your doctor. (No sunscreen until four weeks post-op.)

No exercise until three weeks post-op. Do not wash your hair until four days after surgery.

THE RECOVERY PERIOD

Be prepared to have some serious swelling. It simply cannot be avoided and is just one step of the recovery process you'll have to endure and pass through.

Once the peel has completed, your new skin will be reddish pink. That color usually doesn't fade out for another six to eight weeks. However, the pinkness can be successfully camouflaged with makeup.

Most people experience a dryness to the skin for several months following the peel, but this is easily corrected with the use of the appropriate products.

Stay out of the sun until the pink color is completely faded. Skin that has been phenol-peeled is not likely to tan well, and since sun-tanning is probably one of the factors that caused your skin to age prematurely, you'll want to avoid sunbathing in general.

PROBLEM SIGNS

Any skin eruptions must be reported immediately. The eruptions could indicate a drug allergy.

Any permanent brown discoloration would normally appear between the fourth and eighth weeks post-op. Stay calm. There are terrific rescue techniques such as creams containing steroids, bleach and Retin-A, that can almost always completely correct the discoloration.

Your biggest responsibility in relation to possible problems is the search and detection of any hard areas under the skin. The hard (knotty) areas could become scars, and scarring is the most serious risk you'll run into with any medium to deep peel. Scars usually develop between the eighth and twelfth weeks post-op. Examine yourself carefully and often for these hard areas, and if you discover any, *report them to your doctor immediately.* These areas are treatable, but the longer you wait, the more likely they are to become scars.

MAKEUP TRICKS

Once the brownish-red soft crust has peeled off completely, wait 48 hours before applying any makeup over your fresh reddish-pink skin. Sometimes a green stick cream (Physicians Formula) is useful to help block out the pink. Usually the appropriate color (to match your neck) of Dermablend, Clinique Continuous Coverage or even a heavier application of any cream foundation previously mentioned will do the trick. Be sure you have moisturizer under the makeup, and dust a few grains of loose powder over the foundation to set it.

CHAPTER TWENTY

Lasers

• • •

The word laser is actually an acronym for Light Amplification by Stimulated Emission of Radiation. Your most important job as a patient is to research and select a doctor who knows as much as possible about this complex field. If it were me, I'd find a dermatologist who's head of the laser department at a hospital or a doctor who's had some papers and articles published on the subject of lasers.

There are many different types of lasers—too many for me to address in this book. Two types are used to treat vascular lesions such as broken blood vessels and port wine stains. One is the pulsed laser, specifically the Candela laser and the Cynasure laser. The other is the continuous wave laser, such as the copper vapor laser, KTP laser, krypton laser, copper bromide laser, argon laser and argon dye laser.

With continuous wave lasers you will have no bruising. The downside is that you'll run a higher risk of pigment loss (being left lighter than your normal skin tone) and texture changes.

Your laser choices will depend on your physical circumstances: the location of the problem, your skin color and quality and your age.

In general, the fairer the skin, the less risk of pigmentation complications. Hyperpigmentation (splotchy darkening of skin color) is more likely to occur in dark-skinned people.

The possible permanent dangers with lasers are basically the same as those with dermabrasion and chemical peels: scarring, discoloration and texture change of the skin.

BROKEN BLOOD VESSELS / APPROXIMATE COST: $200–$800 *depending on size of the areas being treated*

APPROXIMATE TIME UNTIL COMPLETELY HEALED:

Five to seven days for actual healing. Residue pinkness could take a few weeks to completely fade out.

BEFORE YOU SET A DATE

With the continuous wave laser, your goal is to completely blanch out the broken blood vessels. With the pulsed lasers, you'll experience some degree of bruising over the corrected area that will fade out in time. Sometimes the blood vessels won't disappear completely, but will fade in color to a large degree.

PREPROCEDURE INSTRUCTIONS

None. Just show up for your appointment.

THE PROCEDURE

Anesthesia is not usually required for treatment of broken blood vessels. However, if your doctor feels you may need numbing, a topical cream called EMLA Creme is applied 45 minutes to an hour prior to the procedure.

For a facial laser procedure you'll be asked to wear protective goggles over your eyes to prevent retinal damage. You'll be placed in a seated or lying position. The procedure can take anywhere from 2 to 20 minutes, depending on the size of the area of broken vessels.

The sensation you'll feel as you're being lasered will be similar to a mild burning or the snapping of a rubber band against the skin. It's not all that uncomfortable.

THE RECOVERY PERIOD

With continuous wave laser systems, healing will involve mild scabbing or crusting that will pass in five to seven days. With the pulsed laser system, you will experience a bruised area, with occasional mild scaling or flaking. This will also pass in five to seven days.

Antibiotic ointment is applied to the area once a day until the healing is complete.

The discomfort is minimal. Sometimes patients are given a dose of Tylenol for the first day, but it's usually not necessary.

PROBLEM SIGNS

For both the continuous wave laser systems and the pulsed system, problem signs would be extensive scabbing, signs of infection and delayed healing (meaning if you're not healed within 10 days, you've got a problem and you will need to see your doctor immediately.)

MAKEUP TRICKS

Do not put makeup on open, blistering or oozing skin. Most patients will experience dry and unbroken skin with pulsed lasers. In these cases patients are encouraged to cover their bruising from the first day of the procedure. This is because the bruising from the pulsed laser system is so dark the first couple of days, you'll require camouflage makeup—and even then, these dark bruises can bleed through the makeup as a gray tone until they begin to fade.

You can use any of the heavier camouflage makeups, such as Clinique Continuous Coverage, Cover Mark, Natural Cover or Dermablend. Apply the heavier coverage makeup directly over your own foundation by patting the camouflage cream over the bruise until the color disappears. Don't forget to lightly powder over the camouflage makeup for longer coverage.

Be extremely careful when removing your makeup after laser procedures until you're completely healed. If you rub too hard, you could accidentally create permanent texture changes in the skin. I recommend that you be very gentle in removing makeup and cleansing for a good three to four weeks post-procedure.

PORT WINE STAINS / APPROXIMATE COST: $200–$1,500
depending on size of the areas being treated

APPROXIMATE TIME UNTIL COMPLETELY HEALED:

Five to seven days for actual healing. Residue pinkness could take a few weeks to completely fade.

BEFORE YOU SET A DATE

Port wine stains are a condition present at birth. The deep wine-colored patches range in size from very small to big enough to cover large portions of the body (in extreme cases). Port wine stains can create enormous self-consciousness in a person, severely damaging his or her self-image. Many people with large port wine stains report that they feel disfigured and embarrassed. The good news is that laser treatment can really help erase port wine stains. The therapy requires multiple treatments, each given at two-to-three-month intervals.

Usually five or six treatments will accomplish significant lightening. However, depending on the actual problem, some people will continue to benefit by up to 15 and 20 treatments.

The pulsed dye laser is the treatment of choice for children with port wine stains.

PREPROCEDURE INSTRUCTIONS

Show up one hour before the procedure for applications of EMLA anesthetic cream.

THE PROCEDURE

You will be asked to wear protective goggles over your eyes to prevent retinal damage, and you'll be placed in a seated or lying position for the actual procedure.

You'll feel mild burning or a sensation that resembles a snapping rubber band against the skin. The procedure can take from 2 to 30 minutes, depending on the size of the area.

THE RECOVERY PERIOD

With continuous wave laser systems, healing will involve mild scabbing or crusting that will pass in five to seven days. With the pulsed laser system, you will probably experience a bruised area, with some mild scaling or flaking. This will also pass in approximately five to seven days. Antibiotic ointment must be applied to the area once a day until the healing is complete.

The discomfort is minimal. Sometimes patients are given a dose of Tylenol, but it's usually not necessary.

PROBLEM SIGNS

For both the continuous wave laser systems and the pulsed system, problem signs would be extensive scabbing, signs of infection and delayed healing (meaning if you're not healed within 10 days, you've got a problem and you will need to see your doctor immediately).

MAKEUP TRICKS

Do not put makeup on open, blistering, or oozing skin. Most patients will experience dry and unbroken skin. In these cases patients are encouraged to cover their bruising from the first day of the procedure. This is because the bruising from the pulsed laser system is so dark the first couple of days that you'll require camouflage makeup—and even then, these dark bruises can bleed through the makeup as a gray tone until they begin to fade.

You can use any of the heavier camouflage makeups such as Clinique Continuous Coverage, Cover Mark, Natural Cover and Dermablend. Apply the heavier coverage makeup directly over your own foundation, and don't forget to lightly powder over the camouflage makeup for longer coverage.

Be extremely careful when removing your makeup after laser procedures until you're completely healed. If you rub too hard, you could accidentally create permanent texture changes in the skin. I recommend that you be very gentle in removing makeup and cleansing for a good three to four weeks post-procedure.

HYPERPIGMENTATION (AGE SPOTS, LIVER SPOTS, SUN SPOTS) / APPROXIMATE COST: $200–$800 *depending on size of the areas being treated.*

APPROXIMATE TIME UNTIL COMPLETELY HEALED:

Five to seven days for actual healing. Residue pinkness could take a few weeks to completely fade.

BEFORE YOU SET A DATE

Your goal is to eliminate the color from age spots, liver spots and sun spots. The spots usually take only one or two treatments to disappear. Some spots may lighten but never totally vanish. "Cafe au lait" spots are tricky: only about half of them will disappear with laser treatment. The danger is that the half that don't respond may actually darken with the procedure. Therefore, be very sure that your doctor pretests a small area before going ahead with any laser treatment.

If your test is OK, your spots will usually disappear in a couple of treatments given at two month intervals.

Pulse system lasers are preferred to correct hyperpigmentation. These lasers are the Q Switched Nd: Yag laser, the Q Switched Ruby laser and the Alexandrite laser.

These three lasers are designed to emit very high power at short intervals, and they have wavelengths that are geared to be absorbed specifically by pigmentation. In other words, the procedure will lighten your spots.

Continuous wave lasers (such as copper vapor) can be used for pigment lesions but are not as specific and present a higher risk of scarring.

PREPROCEDURE INSTRUCTIONS

If your doctor feels you require a topical anesthetic, arrive at the office for your appointment one hour prior to the procedure for application of EMLA Creme.

THE PROCEDURE

For a facial laser procedure, you'll be asked to wear protective goggles over your eyes to prevent retinal damage. You'll be placed in a seated or lying position. The procedure can take anywhere from 2 to 20 minutes, depending on the size of the spots to be removed. The sensation you'll feel as you're being lasered will be similar to a mild burning or the snapping of a rubber band against the skin.

THE RECOVERY PERIOD

Expect some scaling. Also expect darkening and discoloration of the area for up to 10 days post-procedure. Bruising and a small amount of blistering can occur and will disappear in approximately 10 days, but count on approximately 10 to 14 days for hands, arms and legs to clear up.

With continuous wave laser systems, healing will involve mild scabbing or crusting that will pass in approximately five to seven days. With the pulsed laser system, you will probably experience a bruised area, with some mild scaling or flaking. This will also pass in approximately five to seven days. Antibiotic ointment needs to be applied to the area once a day until the healing is complete.

The discomfort is minimal. Sometimes patients are given a dose of Tylenol, but it's usually not necessary.

PROBLEM SIGNS

For both the continuous wave laser systems and the pulsed system, problem signs would be extensive scabbing, signs of infection and delayed healing (meaning if you're not healed within 10 days, you've got a problem and your doctor needs to see you immediately).

MAKEUP TRICKS

Do not put makeup on open, blistering or oozing skin. Most patients will experience dry and unbroken skin. In these cases patients are encouraged to cover their bruising from the first day of the procedure. This is because the bruising from the pulsed laser system is so dark the first couple of days that you'll require camouflage makeup—and even then, these dark bruises can bleed through the makeup as a gray tone until they begin to fade.

You can use any of the heavier camouflage makeups such as Clinique Continuous Coverage, Cover Mark, Natural Cover and

Dermablend. Apply the heavier coverage makeup directly over your own foundation by patting the camouflage cream over the bruise until the color disappears. Lightly powder over the camouflage makeup for longer coverage.

Be extremely careful when removing your makeup after laser procedures until you're completely healed. If you rub too hard, you could accidentally create permanent texture changes in the skin. Being careful with your makeup removal and cleansing for a good three to four weeks post-procedure is a must!

TATTOO REMOVAL / APPROXIMATE COST: $200–$800
depending on size of the areas being treated

APPROXIMATE TIME UNTIL COMPLETELY HEALED:

Seven days for actual healing. The tattoo will continue to fade over the next three months.

BEFORE YOU SET A DATE

Your goal is to remove all the color from the tattoo. Pulse system lasers are used for tattoo removal: the Alexandrite or Ruby laser removes black, blue and green ink, and the Q Switched Nd: Yag laser removes red, blue and black ink. Flesh- and rouge-colored inks may turn black with the laser and should be pretested prior to full laser treatment.

Tattoo removal usually takes five or six laser treatments given at two-month intervals. Amateur tattoos that involve less ink can disappear in three or four sessions. Not all tattoos will disappear completely, but they will fade considerably.

PREPROCEDURE INSTRUCTIONS

Tattoo removal with the Ruby, the Nd: Yag or the Alexandrite laser can be quite painful, and local anesthesia is definitely suggested. If using EMLA Creme, be sure you're at the doctor's office 1 hour prior to the procedure so that you have several applications of EMLA Creme before lasering. This usually neutralizes serious pain very effectively. If you prefer, you can apply EMLA at home and arrive to your appointment at the procedure time.

THE PROCEDURE

You will be seated or in a lying position. The actual procedure will take anywhere from 1 to 30 minutes, depending on the size of the tattoo.

THE RECOVERY PERIOD

If the Alexandrite or Ruby laser was used, you can expect some swelling and blisters that will heal in seven to ten days.

The healing with the Q Switched Nd: Yag laser is a little less traumatic. Expect some mild scaling that will probably disappear in a week.

A topical antibiotic on the area should be applied twice a day. The area will be bandaged and the dressing must also be changed twice daily until it's totally healed.

If the Q Switched Nd: Yag laser was used to remove only red, you'll probably need to bandage for only a couple of days.

Limited postprocedure activity can minimize the possibility of permanent scarring. You need to discuss this subject with your doctor before leaving the office. A follow-up office visit usually occurs four to six weeks after the procedure.

PROBLEM SIGNS

With the pulsed lasers, problem signs would be extensive scabbing, any signs of infection and delayed healing (meaning if you're not healed within 10 days, you've got a problem and you need to see your doctor immediately).

MAKEUP TRICKS

Do not put makeup on open, blistering or oozing skin. You'll be using only your antibiotic ointments.

CHAPTER TWENTY ONE

Laser Skin Resurfacing

• • •

APPROXIMATE COST:

Full Face: $2,500–$7,000

Eyes: $800–$1,500

Full Mouth: $800–$1,500

Upper Lip Only: $400–$750

APPROXIMATE TIME UNTIL COMPLETELY HEALED:

It normally takes 8 to 10 days for the newly lasered skin to completely heal.

The bright pink color usually takes six to eight weeks to fade out, but some people have experienced the pinkness for up to eight months post-laser. It could take up to several months to fade completely.

BEFORE YOU SET A DATE

Laser resurfacing is successfully being used to improve sun-damaged skin, facial wrinkles, scarring and acne scars. The laser has a few advantages over dermabrasion and chemical peels because it is a relatively (if not completely) bloodless procedure and is much neater and cleaner than dermabrasion. Dermabrasion can very often create loss of pigment, leaving the patient with permanent white areas on the skin. Lasers present a lower risk for this type of pigment loss because they're computerized for depth control and have a precise release time of short, concentrated exposures of light that can be monitored in a very controlled manner.

If your doctor is concerned about pigment alteration due to your skin type (olive skin is especially susceptible), he may choose to pretest a small area of your facial skin.

If you've taken an acne treatment called Isotretinoin within the past year, forget any thought of laser treatment! You may not heal properly. Make absolutely sure you discuss this with your doctor.

Lasering the face will improve most wrinkles and tighten the skin up considerably. In some cases, this may be all that the patient needs. But it doesn't always take the place of a face-lift, particularly if your facial muscles require tightening. For wrinkle removal, the areas around the eyes and the mouth seem to respond the best.

Significant improvement can be seen when the entire face is resurfaced. Doing your full face as opposed to lasering only specific areas increases the likelihood that your new skin texture will match over the entire face. But don't worry—if you only want to remove the wrinkles and tighten the area around the eye, you'll probably be quite happy with the end result.

The laugh lines that run from the sides of your nostrils to the corners of your mouth won't show too much improvement with skin resurfacing unless you laser the entire face. The general tightening of the face can improve the appearance of deep laugh lines in the same way a face-lift would tighten that laugh line area.

There are two types of lasers used for skin resurfacing: the Silk Touch Scanner laser and the Ultrapulse CO_2 laser. Both lasers offer similar results. The choice of laser is entirely up to your doctor.

The laser usually takes one to four passes over the skin to significantly improve wrinkles. The number of laser passes varies depending on the site. For instance, the eyelids require much less due to the thinness of the skin.

With luck, you can expect a 50 percent wrinkle improvement after one laser treatment. Acne scars will improve about 25 percent with the first treatment, depending on the type of scar. Many people opt for a repeat treatment for maximum results.

The lasered areas will ooze for the first four to seven days after lasering, so prepare yourself for a week's worth of messy lubricating and soaking. Believe me, you're going to want to hide out at home for the first week at least, so don't plan any public outings!

PREPROCEDURE INSTRUCTIONS

Lasering is always easier on fairer skin because there is less risk of pigmentation problems. This also holds true with any chemical peel or dermabrasion. However, for all types of skin, special preparation must be carefully prescribed and followed two to four weeks before lasering. If you have slightly darker-toned skin, you'll need to use a prescription bleach such as Melenex for two weeks prior to the procedure.

If you are Asian or Hispanic, the lasering must be done with a little more caution to protect against pigment alterations. Special pre- and postprocedure care is used for Asian and Hispanic skin. Asians and Hispanics will use Retin-A, bleach creams, kogic acid and/or hydroquinones at least two to four weeks before lasering. They will resume these treatments one month post laser and continue them for perhaps several months.

1. You will be instructed to use a special prescription pre-procedure cream (Retin-A 0.1%, hydroquinone 5% and desonide 0.1%) every night two to four weeks prior to the laser treatment.

2. Each morning you must use a broad-spectrum sunscreen.

3. You'll need to wash your face only with soap-free cleaners (Aquanil or Cetaphil).

4. You'll be given antibiotic pills to start the day before or the day of the laser treatment.

5. You'll be given a Zovirax pill to take the day before or the day of treatment to protect against any possible herpes eruptions.

Patients who are not Asian or Hispanic will be instructed to:
1. Apply a daily morning broad-spectrum sunscreen along with a prescription cream of hydroquinone (2% hydroquinone cream, 10% glycolic acid gel, or 4% hydroquinone liquid or cream).

2. Apply Retin-A cream 0.025% or 0.05% every night for two to four weeks prior to the laser procedure.

3. Wash your face with a soap-free cleanser only (Aquanil or Cetaphil).

4. Take an antibiotic pill the day before or the day of the laser procedure.

5. Take a Zovirax pill the day before or the day of the procedure to protect against possible herpes outbreak.

THE PROCEDURE

Arrive an hour and a half prior to the actual laser treatment for applications of topical EMLA anesthetic cream. Extrasensitive patients will probably need some local injections of anesthesia.

You will be placed in a lying position and given protective goggles for your eyes. If you're having your eyes done, you'll be given special contact lenses to prevent retinal damage.

With the new laser equipment, the actual procedure takes only about 30 to 40 minutes for full-face resurfacing and 15 minutes for the eyes. The mouth area usually requires only 15 minutes.

As the laser passes over the area of treatment, you might feel a mild burning sensation.

When you sit up and look at yourself you'll be rather swollen, and you'll see a dry white, yellowish or pinkish tone to your skin. Your skin will feel as though you have a fresh sunburn.

Vigilon, a wet, gel-based dressing, will be applied to the lasered area for your first 24 hours post-procedure.

The next day you'll remove the dressing and start lubricating the lasered skin six times a day with Crisco vegetable shortening. Yes, that's right. I said Crisco. It's used as a lubricant because it does the job and doesn't produce allergic irritations on post-lasered skin the way many antibiotic ointments do. The lasered area must remain extremely lubricated for seven days following the procedure. The lubrication will help eliminate that tight, itchy uncomfortable feeling. It's also essential to proper healing, so whatever you do, make sure you smear that Crisco on six times a day.

Obviously you're going to want to sleep on an old pillowcase that you don't care about keeping after your seven days of Crisco! Some patients prefer to wear the Vigilon dressing through the night so they don't run the risk of drying out.

POSTPROCEDURE INSTRUCTIONS
DAY ONE:

1. You will be wearing your wet dressing over the lasered skin.

2. Take your antibiotic medication as instructed.

3. Take your Zovirax medication as instructed.

4. If you need a painkiller, you're given Tylenol with codeine for the first couple of days. Many people don't need any pain medication at all.

DAYS TWO OR THREE:

1. You should be checked by your doctor in the office the day following the laser treatment. Follow-up office checks usually continue every three days until you've normalized.

2. Gently remove your wet dressing.

3. Dip a clean washcloth or soft paper towels in ice water and soak the lasered skin for 7 to 10 minutes, three or four times a day. Make it easy on yourself and schedule the ice-water soaks before breakfast, lunch, dinner and bedtime. You must use a fresh, clean washcloth or paper towel at each of these four separate ice-water soakings. Do not reuse the same towels or cloths. You don't want to give yourself an infection.

4. Sometime in the afternoon, between lunch and dinner, you'll need to give yourself another 7-to-10-minute soak. This time it's an acetic soak, meaning that you need to mix one capful of distilled white vinegar in two cups of ice water, and once again soak with clean towels.

    This particular acetic soak is very important because it will cut down on the oozing. So don't forget to do this every day for seven days post-procedure.

5. Between all these soakings, you absolutely must continue to smear that Crisco on the lasered areas at least six times a day.

DAYS FOUR THROUGH SEVEN:

1. Continue antibiotic medication as instructed.

2. Continue Zovirax as instructed.

3. Continue your ice-water and acetic soaks.

4. Continue to apply Crisco six times a day.

5. If any irritation develops you'll be given a cortisone ointment to apply to specific areas as instructed by your doctor.

6. If your swelling hasn't normalized by the end of your fifth day post-laser, call your doctor and schedule an office visit. As mentioned before, you should be having office follow-ups every three days until you've healed, no matter what.

WEEKS TWO AND THREE:

1. Wash with a soap-free cleanser (Aquanil or Cetaphil).

2. Your doctor will give you titanium dioxide containing sunscreen (Neutropenia SPF 17) to apply daily.

WEEK FOUR:

1. Apply a broad-spectrum sunscreen every day. Discuss the sunscreen choices with your doctor.

2. Apply Retin-A cream 0.025% or 0.05% every night.

3. You'll be given topical hydroquinone to be applied every morning. (If darkening of the skin has occurred, ask your doctor about giving you a 2% hydroquinone, 10% glycolic acid gel.)

4. Continue to wash daily with your soap-free cleanser (Aquanil or Cetaphil).

THE RECOVERY PERIOD

As I mentioned before, you'll definitely want to hide out for the first week.

It's imperative that you follow all of your post-laser care to the last detail. Give yourself all the help you can to achieve the best possible healing. As with all peels, you must stay out of the sun for at least two months to avoid permanent darkening on your new skin. Wear a hat when you go out.

After you go through laser skin resurfacing, any doctor will advise you to stay out of the sun for the rest of your life. The lasering has removed years from your skin and given you a new chance to be smart: No more sunbathing. Never again! That's one of your most important factors in keeping your skin healthy and beautiful.

PROBLEM SIGNS

Any signs of possible infection or excessive pain would require an immediate call to your doctor. Also, if your healing has not completed within 10 days, you'll need to schedule an appointment.

MAKEUP TRICKS

Makeup must never be applied until at least 7 to 10 days post-laser, and do not apply any makeup over broken or oozing skin.

Apply your moisturizer before your foundation. Your face will be bright pink, so you'll have to find your appropriate color by matching your makeup skin color to your neck or upper chest. Cream foundations will give more complete coverage during your next weeks of bright pinkness. Dermablend, Cover Mark, Clinique Continuous Coverage or a heavier application of any cream foundations mentioned previously will do the trick.

Be sure to dust a few grains of loose powder over the foundation to set it. Apply the powder with a soft brush. If you use a powder puff it will look too heavy on the skin.

Be extremely careful when removing your makeup after laser procedures. If you rub too hard, you could create permanent texture changes in the skin. I recommend that you be very gentle when removing makeup and cleansing for a month post-procedure.

CHAPTER TWENTY TWO

Collagen, Fat Injections and Silicone

. . .

COLLAGEN / APPROXIMATE COST: $150–$400 *each visit.*

Collagen is sold by the syringe. The smaller syringes are used for fine lines and small area touch-ups. The larger syringes are used for full-face treatment.

Collagen is a natural protein that pads and offers structure to the skin as well as to ligaments, bones and other parts of the body. As you age, this padding under your skin wears down, leaving you with wrinkles and lines.

Injectable collagen is a natural protein made from purified cow collagen. Two types of collagen are available: Zyderm, which is a lighter form of collagen and is used mainly for superficial lines like those around the lips and eyes; and Zyplast, which is more effective for deeper correction such as laugh and frown lines.

Zyplast collagen usually requires only one visit to achieve desired results. In contrast, Zyderm needs to be built up over time—you'll make several visits three or four weeks apart to attain the complete effect. These multiple visits will cost you a bit more, but that's the nature of working with Zyderm.

Collagen is useful for smoothing facial wrinkles, correcting contour deformities and modifying many types of scars. Acne scars respond particularly well to collagen injections, whereas scars with well-defined edges are not likely to be helped by collagen.

Although many women have used collagen injections to enlarge the size of their lips, this treatment is not a recommended procedure; there are too many muscles in the lips that could be injured.

Prior to a collagen treatment you'll have to undergo a skin test to determine if you're sensitive to the product. A pea-sized drop is injected into the underside of your forearm, and allergic reactions are usually obvious over the next four weeks. If the spot swells, becomes red and itches, you are not a candidate for collagen. Occasionally someone can have a compatible skin test and still be allergic to the collagen. This happened to me, and I didn't discover the allergy until the collagen was in my face. I had injected it to plump out two very small vertical lines above my upper lip. Two months after the injection, I would swell up violently in those two spots when I was premenstrual. The problem required monthly medication and injections of steroids until the collagen finally disappeared from my body.

Allergic reactions to collagen can produce prolonged swelling, redness, hardness, itching and even cysts that become hard and may permanently scar. The good news for allergy sufferers is that injectable collagen is not a permanent fixture in your body. It dissolves in three months to a year, finally eliminating your problem. The other downside to prolonged use of collagen is the possibility of needle damage to skin that is injected in the same area over and over again.

Lately, there has been a great deal of media coverage linking collagen injections to autoimmune diseases, specifically rheumatoid arthritis, lupus, and polymyositis/dermatomyositis (PM/DM—two extremely rare autoimmune diseases that involve destruction of muscle tissues). The truth is that medical experts are unable to determine any precise cause or cure for most autoimmune diseases. This means that there is no specific current research data to confirm or refute the idea that collagen is linked to autoimmune disease. However, be very clear about the following statement: If you do have an autoimmune disease such as rheumatoid arthritis or lupus, do not use collagen or fibril, because you could be hypersensitive to it.

Like everything else discussed in this book, collagen injections involve some degree of risk. In fact, there are doctors in Texas who believe the risk can be quite serious. Nevertheless, many people find that these injections do successfully and safely plump out their lines, wrinkles and flaws and make them look considerably younger.

Other line-fillers are still being perfected. One is Plasmagel, an injection derived by separating out the protein-rich plasma from the patient's own blood. Gore-Tex is the only line filler that isn't administered with a needle. Gore-Tex is actually a fabric that's cut into fine strips and placed under the skin with a small tube. The tiny incision lines at either end of the Gore-Tex strip will probably be sutured for 24 hours and should heal easily with minimum visual consequences.

The consensus seems to be that the line-filler of the future is a product called Hylan B Gel. This product is a form of hyaluronic acid, which is a natural component of the skin. Hylan B Gel doesn't require a skin test. Apparently no one has been allergic to Hylan B Gel to date. As with most line-fillers, you can expect to experience some redness and swelling for a day or so following the injection, but it will disappear. Hylan B Gel is still awaiting FDA approval and isn't available as yet. Too bad—it appears to be safe and effective.

Botox (botulinim toxin) is not a line-filler. It temporarily paralyzes the individual muscles that form expression lines across the forehead and around the eyes. Patients under 50 years of age seem to receive the most benefit from Botox, because younger skin is usually thicker and more responsive.

In the Botox treatment, small amounts of dilute concentrations of Botox are injected into the specific sites. Paralyzing effects last only three to six months, and then you'll need to repeat the procedure. The FDA has not approved Botox as a cosmetic line-corrector, but it has been approved in treating muscle twitching around the eyes. Nonetheless, some patients are opting for Botox injections as a cosmetic line-corrector. The injections should be monitored through an electromyograph, which allows the doctor to locate the most electrically active portion of the muscle.

Be very clear about one thing: Botox is to be used only in the upper third portion of the face. Injections of Botox elsewhere on the face could cause droopy lips and even prevent your face muscles from functioning.

Removing a small amount of your own body fat and depositing that fat into another area is the only 100 percent sure bet that you will never have an allergic reaction to the transplant. You cannot develop an allergy to your own body fat.

These fat injections have become extremely popular for correcting contour deformities and in plumping out certain areas cosmetically. However, don't confuse fat injections with collagen injections, silicone droplets or bio-plastique: fat will work only in certain areas and is not recommended for cosmetic purposes such as plumping out the fine lines around the mouth and eyes. Fat is generally used for deeper implanting than collagen; it would tend to lump up and look uneven if it were injected superficially as collagen is.

The fat is generally removed from your stomach or your buttocks. The area is first numbed up locally with injections of Xylocaine, and then a large 18-gauge needle is introduced into the anesthetized site and a small amount of fat is abstracted into the syringe. Don't be alarmed by the size of the needle. You won't feel any pain—just a pumping sensation as the fat is being sucked into the syringe. However, if a blood vessel is accidentally hit by the 18-gauge needle, you'll definitely feel it, so you may want to be given a general "twilight" anesthesia that will greatly reduce your awareness.

The next step is for the doctor to locally anesthetize the area of your face that will receive the fat, unless you've been given a "twilight," in which case local anesthesia is unnecessary. Certain areas, such as the cheeks, are apparently too painful to work on even with a local anesthetic, so most doctors insist on a brief general anesthetic in treating those areas.

The needle is introduced into the appropriate site and the fat is injected. Expect some temporary bruising and swelling. Depending on the site, the procedure may need to be repeated more than once to achieve the desired results.

The main risk about fat injections is simply that they might not work. Some people's bodies don't accept the fat transplant and it is absorbed by the body. However, if your body accepts the transplanted fat, it can last in the site for many years before needing to be reinjected. There's really no way to gauge how your body will respond.

Many doctors are using fat for lip enlargement. In my opinion, it usually looks terrible, leaving the patient with Donald Duck lips.

I've not seen many fat-injected lips that look natural, and because of this I don't personally recommend this procedure.

SILICONE

The only remark I can conscientiously make about large amounts of liquid silicone being injected into the face or body is: Never do it! I am talking about liquid silicone injections, not to be confused with silicone implants, which are an entirely different subject.

The injection of liquid silicone into the body was studied by a group of dermatologists and plastic surgeons for a number of years and has never been approved as a medical technique. Although liquid silicone injections are not illegal, they are not a widely accepted medical approach. Most plastic surgeons feel that the injection of silicone into the tissues is inappropriate because of the lack of control the doctor has over the material (large injected amounts can end up drifting all over your body), as well as the high incidents of formation of inflammatory tissue to the silicone.

Liquid silicone injections are a highly controversial subject. Many doctors have different opinions regarding the subject and the consensus is that *the amount of silicone injected into the body is directly related to the risk.*

For example, some doctors are injecting silicone microdroplets into the face to plump out depressed areas and lines. The procedure is done very gradually, a single droplet at a time. If the area requires only a limited number of droplets to correct the problem, the risk remains minimal. Many people have no bad side effects at all.

Some patients experience temporary swelling in the silicone-injected area, the same type of swelling that can occur with collagen. In a very few cases, the droplet may turn hard and require injecting with triamcinolone acetonide, shaving, or dermabrasion.

Bioplastique is another form of injectable silicone. Here the silicone particles are even smaller than in the microdroplet procedure. This procedure has been used by doctors in Europe for several years now, with mostly positive results.

The truth is, everyone reacts differently to foreign objects introduced into the body. Some people experience reactions, while others sail through with no problems. As for the long-term side effects of injecting micro amounts of silicone, most doctors believe it to be safe, but to date no scientific data exists on the topic.

Afterword

...

As with all medical procedures and techniques, science is making continual progress, and improved techniques will be introduced as practiced by surgeons. As these advancements occur and become safe and approved medical procedures, this book will be updated to include new information and fee updates.

I have tried to educate the reader that elective plastic surgery is not a superficial event. My intent has been to inform and prepare the patient for the medical, emotional and psychological realities of the surgery they are contemplating.

I do hope that this has been of help.

—*Diana Barry*
January 1996

Index

• • •

Page numbers in *italics* refer to illustrations in the text.

eye makeup, 44-46, *47*

F

face-lift
  appearance immediately following, 20
  endoscopic, 81
  fantasies about results of, 13
  good reasons for, 13
  healing time, 14
  helmet dressings, 24, 31
  judging results of, 14, 34-35
  as major surgical procedure, 19
  perfection not achieved by, 14, 15
  recovery time, 19-20
  trade-offs, 14, 15
face-lift, lower, 27-32, *30-32*
  cost, approximate, 27
  steps in, 28-29
  surgical procedure, 27-29
facial-line fillers, 181-183
facial peel, deep (phenol), 157-161
  considerations, 158
  cosmetic camouflage, 161
  cost, approximate, 157
  postprocedure instructions, 159-160
  preprocedure instructions, 159
  problem signs, 161
  procedure, 159
  recovery period, 160-161
  results and trade-offs, 157-158
  time until healed, 157
facial peel, light (glycolic acid), 149-151
  benefits of, 149
  cost, approximate, 149
  moisturizing following peel, 151
  preprocedure instructions, 150
  problem signs, 151
  procedure, 150
  recovery period, 151
facial peel, medium (TCA)
  best candidates for, 155
  cost, approximate, 152
  moisturizing after, 156
  postprocedure instructions, 154
  preprocedure instructions, 152-153
  problem signs, 155
  procedure, 153-154
  recovery period, 154-155
  time until healed, 152
facial skin, laser resurfacing. *See* laser skin
  resurfacing
fatigue after plastic surgery, 14, 19-20, 33,
  40
fat injections, 184-185
  cost, approximate, 184
  risks, 184
forehead-lift. *See* brow- and coronal-lifts

G

girdle, surgical, *128*
Gore-Tex strips, 183

H

hair, 39-40
  loss after coronal surgery, 78
  preparation for coronal surgery, 76
healing time. *See under type of procedure
  or surgery*
heating pads, avoiding, 38
helmet dressings, 24, 31
herpes, 175
homeopathic remedies, 21-22
Hylan B Gel, 183
hyperpigmentation, laser treatment of, 168-
170

I

ice applications, 38, 54
implants
  breast, 83, 85-90, *91-93*
  calf, 146, *148*
  cheek, 139-142
  chin, 141-145, *147*
  nasal, 64
  pectoral, 146
incisions/incision lines, 55
  for abdominoplasty, 131, 132, *135*
  avoiding sun on, 37
  for breast augmentation, 88, *91*
  for brow- and coronal-lifts, 75, *79*
  for brow-lift, 74-75
  for chin implants, 144
  for coronal lifts, 75
  at ears, painful, 39
  for endoscopic surgery, 82, 83
  for eyelid surgery, 53
  healing process, 35-36
  for liposuction, 123-124, *127*
  for lower face-lift, *30*
  in lower face-lift, 29-29
  makeup and, 41
  oozing from, 55
  in post-mastectomy reconstruction, 111
  rhinoplasty, 63, 64

J

jaw, removal of fat beneath, 28

K

keloids, 90, 98

L

lasers, 163-171
  continuous wave, 163, 168
  pulse system, 163, 168, 170
  types of, 163, 168, 174

for liposuction, 122
for rhinoplasty, 62-63
presurgical period, 20
  homeopathic remedies in, 21-22
  vitamin and mineral supplements during,
    22

R
recovery period, 33-40
  for abdominoplasty, 133-134
  after face-lift, 14, 19-20
  after medium facial peel, 154-155
  appearance during, 33-36
  for breast augmentation, 89, 98
  for brow- and coronal-lifts, 77-78
  for cheek implants, 142
  for chin implants, 145
  depression in, 36
  for eyelid surgery, 54-55
  getting back to normal, 37-38
  for laser skin resurfacing, 178-179
  for liposuction, 125-126
  normal sensations during, 38-40
  for post-mastectomy reconstruction, 114
  for rhinoplasty, 65-66
  touch-ups and, 15
rhinoplasty, 61-71
  anesthesia for, 63
  consultations preceding, 61
  cosmetic camouflage of, 67
  cost, approximate, 61
  incisions, *68*
  incisions for, *63*
  nasal implants, 64
  nasal packing, 65, *70*
  open, 63
  postsurgical instructions, 64-65
  presurgical instructions, 62-63
  problem signs, 66-67
  receding chin and, 62
  recovery period, 65-66
  septum work, 63
  surgical procedures, 63-34, *68-71*
  time until healed, 61
  touch-up surgery after, 66

S
scarring, 90, 98
  after medium facial peel, 155
  herpes and, 150, 153, 158
  from lasers, 163
silicone, liquid, injections of, 185
  warnings and risks, 185
skin
  excess, removal of, 28, 29, 53
  postsurgical, 39
  sloughing after abdominoplasty, 133
skin type, 14

smoking, 52, 62, 74, 87, 96, 110, 130, 143
staples, for coronal-lift, 75-76
steroids, 34, 37
sun, avoiding, 51
sun spots, laser treatment of, 168-170
surgical garments, 124
  girdle, *128*
surgical problems
  correction of, 14-15, 66
surgical procedures
  lower face-lift, 27-29
sutures, cleaning, 37
swelling. *See also* Distorted Period
  after rhinoplasty, 65-66
  following liposuction, 125
  silicone injections and, 185
systemic makeup, 14

T
tattoo removal, 170-171
  types of lasers for, 170, 171
TCA peel. *See* facial peel, medium
tummy tuck. *See* abdominoplasty
Tylenol, 51, 54, 62

V
vitamin C, 22
vitamin E, 22, 97
vitamin K, 22
vitamin supplements, 22

X
Xylocaine, 28, 184

Z
Zovirax, 150, 153, 158, 175, 176
Zyderm collagen, 181
Zyplast collagen, 181